Praise for Alla Svirins

'The high-class healer.'
THE TIMES

'Super-guru of London.'
EVENING STANDARD

'Highly regarded with a waiting list for months.'
THE SUNDAY TELEGRAPH

'Alla is a Russian energy healer who is the talk of three coasts – Hollywood, New York and London.'
VOGUE

'Her famous and famously sceptical patients are a healthy testimony to her extraordinary powers.'
HARPERS & QUEEN

'Alla engenders universal praise from her clients.'
MAIL ON SUNDAY

'Alla is a remarkable practitioner and I consider myself very fortunate to know her.'
SARAH, DUCHESS OF YORK

'An amazing woman who even the most cynical swear by.'
TATLER

'Energy healer to the stars.'
HUFFPOST

'Alla is the healer of the moment.'
WOMAN & HOME

'Remarkable healing powers.'
KINDRED SPIRIT

'The wellness guru people are traveling for.'
CONDÉ NAST TRAVELER

'Alla will take your body and soul on a journey of holistic rejuvenation.'
SPIRIT & DESTINY

'Gifted woman behind the revolutionary treatment of bio-energy balancing.'
GOOD HEALTH

'Alla shows you how to cleanse your entire body inside and out to unleash unique powers of energy, shift the dynamics in your life and give you a detox like no other.
WOMEN'S FITNESS

'Alla Svirinskaya's name is known to every successful and trendy resident of London.'
VOGUE RUSSIA

'Possesses an almost clairvoyant touch... She had the guests at Parrot Cay fighting for an appointment.'
THE SUNDAY TIMES STYLE

'An impressive client list.'
THE SUN

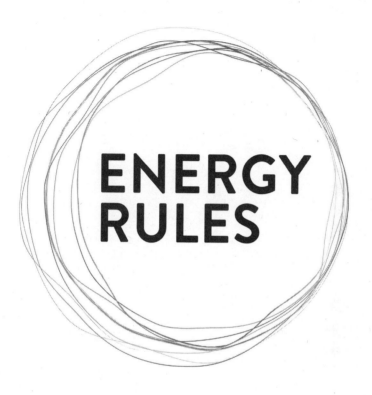

ENERGY RULES

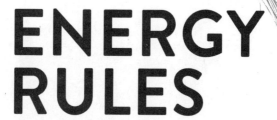

ENERGY RULES

**Deflect Negative
Vibrations and
Own Your Energy**

ALLA SVIRINSKAYA

HAY HOUSE

Carlsbad, California • New York City
London • Sydney • New Delhi

Published in the United Kingdom by:
Hay House UK Ltd, The Sixth Floor, Watson House,
54 Baker Street, London W1U 7BU
Tel: +44 (0)20 3927 7290; Fax: +44 (0)20 3927 7291; www.hayhouse.co.uk

Published in the United States of America by:
Hay House Inc., PO Box 5100, Carlsbad, CA 92018-5100
Tel: (1) 760 431 7695 or (800) 654 5126; Fax: (1) 760 431 6948 or (800) 650 5115
www.hayhouse.com

Published in Australia by:
Hay House Australia Ltd, 18/36 Ralph St, Alexandria NSW 2015
Tel: (61) 2 9669 4299; Fax: (61) 2 9669 4144; www.hayhouse.com.au

Published in India by:
Hay House Publishers India, Muskaan Complex, Plot No.3, B-2,
Vasant Kunj, New Delhi 110 070
Tel: (91) 11 4176 1620; Fax: (91) 11 4176 1630; www.hayhouse.co.in

Text © Alla Svirinskaya, 2019, 2023

Previously published in 2019 as *Own Your Energy*
(tradepaper ISBN: 978-1-78817-298-1)

A catalogue record for this book is available from the British Library.

Tradepaper ISBN: 978-1-4019-7321-6
E-book ISBN: 978-1-78817-951-5
Audiobook ISBN: 978-1-78817-952-2

Interior images: Leanne Siu Anastasi

10 9 8 7 6 5 4 3 2 1

Printed in the United States of America

Dedicated to the Universe with the deepest gratitude, awareness and appreciation.

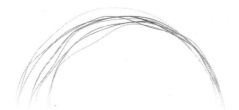

Contents

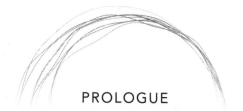

Back to the Future – Hidden Risks to Our Wellbeing

Can you imagine drinking water from a sewerage system while you're recovering from diarrhoea, or kissing a friend who is bed-bound with flu, or having unprotected sex with a partner who has an STD? Such actions seem crazily risky, even dangerous, to us, yet our ancestors wouldn't have thought twice about doing them.

In parts of Europe during the early Enlightenment (1685– 1730), cleaning the body was regarded as 'heathen' because the Bible says that 'He who is once washed in Christ need not wash again.'[1] Some religious leaders interpreted this scripture literally, and taught that taking a bath would dissolve one's association with the Divine. Bathing was regarded as an unchristian thing to do.

Unsurprisingly, then, most people didn't ever wash their bodies, and as a result they suffered from all sorts of skin conditions. Despite the various 'cures' on offer, patients failed to recover from their ailments because they were simply unaware of the correlation between a lack of cleanliness and infection. This and many similarly hazardous practices ensured that in this period, and indeed throughout most of human history, people were caught up in an endless cycle of contracting an infectious disease, attempting a cure, sabotage, and then a recurrence of that disease.

Hostages of the Unseen

Today we're amazed by this level of ignorance and reassure ourselves that our own lives are so much safer and more hygienic. We take daily showers and wash our hands after using the bathroom; we know to use protection to avoid contracting STDs; patients with contagious conditions are quarantined; and generally, we afford all aspects of personal hygiene the utmost priority. In fact, many of us are now so conscious of hygiene that we carry antibacterial sprays and wipes around with us, so we can remove any germs we encounter and exterminate them before they do any harm.

Imagine how our ancestors would react if they could see us doing all these things. They would probably be astonished or, most likely, ridicule us, because until relatively recently, as we're about to discuss, no one was aware that germs even existed. It reminds me of the saying 'And those who were seen dancing were thought to be insane by those who could not hear the music.'

So you might think that there's absolutely no connection between the environment in which our ancestors lived, with bacteria and viruses running riot, and the safe, squeaky-clean world in which we in the West live today. After all, unlike us, our forebears exposed themselves to all manner of health dangers, many times a day in many different ways, and often suffered greatly as a result. They had little idea of even basic hygiene practices, whereas we know exactly how to protect ourselves.

Well, what I'm about to share with you might come as a surprise. Yes, we may be a lot cleaner and much more clued up about how to lead sanitary lives, but many of us are completely unaware that we need to take our personal hygiene *to a whole new level*. By this, I don't mean protecting ourselves from biological pathogens such as viruses, bacteria and fungi. I'm talking about managing the pathogens in the unseen world of energy around us.

Many people don't know that these 'energy pathogens' exist and are therefore oblivious of the numerous ways in which they can affect us. And, just as happened to our ancestors, our ignorance of the existence of these pathogens, and our failure to protect ourselves from them, enables them to contaminate us and seriously compromise our wellbeing.

Having healed thousands of people over the past two decades, I've discovered that exposure to such 'energy toxicity' is one of the main ways in which we sabotage our wellness. Later in the book, we'll explore energy toxicity and I'll describe my concept behind energy pathogens.

The Microscopic Universe

But right now, we're going to take a closer look at how ignorance of the unseen world of germs negatively affected our not-so-distant ancestors. Afterwards, I'll explain how our modern society – which is sophisticated in so many ways – is making the same mistakes about *another* invisible realm. Actually, perhaps these shouldn't be classified as mistakes, but instead as a stage in human evolution from which, thanks to our more advanced understanding of the world and ourselves, we can move to another level.

Even just a few centuries ago, people were unaware of the microbial ecosystem that lives around us, on our skin and inside our bodies: they couldn't see all those hundreds of trillions of bacteria, viruses and other organisms so they didn't know they were there. This meant that no one, not even those in the medical profession, had a clue about the vital role that hygiene plays in preventing the spread of disease-causing pathogens.

People took medicine to rid themselves of an illness but then they'd contract that illness once more. The problem was that they didn't know *how* they'd become unwell in the first place, so they had no idea how to prevent it from happening again. It wasn't until 1665 that English scientist Robert Hooke used a microscope to observe the tiniest, previously hidden details of the natural world, and discovered the first known microbes, including moulds; and it was only in 1675 that Dutchman Antonie van Leeuwenhoek, using a microscope that he'd made himself, discovered the existence of bacteria.

But even after these momentous scientific breakthroughs, the vast majority of the population remained in blissful ignorance of the existence of germs and the harmful effects they can have. As a result they were caught up in that endless cycle of disease and cure I mentioned earlier. A doctor might administer the best medicine of the day (which, from our perspective, isn't saying much!) to treat a violent stomach upset, but it would almost certainly return because if the patient recovered they'd continue eating with dirty hands or consuming rotting food. They'd be back to square one. And so it went on.

Higher Life Versus Lower Life

By the time the 19th century arrived, people were a lot more clued up about the damage that biological pathogens could wreak on the human body. Scientists had acquired a far greater understanding of microbes and their impact on human health. These microbes were called 'house diseases' and 'insidious foes', and were classified as 'the lower life'. Humans, on the other hand, were 'the higher life'. A battle ensued between the two.[2]

Epidemics of cholera and other infectious diseases were rife throughout the 19 century, and people were desperate to protect themselves. It's hard to imagine that a little more than 150 years ago, the medical profession believed in the 'miasmatic' theory, which held that most disease was caused by inhaling foul smells, or 'bad air', arising from decayed organic matter. Until fairly recently, hospital architecture was heavily influenced by miasmatic theory and buildings were designed to allow in as much fresh, clean air as possible.

Public health campaigns – targeted mostly at housewives – emphasized the importance of disease prevention through cleaning. (At first, though, this was about eradicating bad smells from the home rather than killing germs.) Domestic hygiene became the driving force of healthy living, and a symbol of high social status.[3]

Interestingly, in the Victorian era in Britain, personal hygiene regained its connection with morality. While in previous centuries people had thought it morally dubious to give oneself a good scrub in the bath, now it was declared morally dubious not to! Cleanliness was definitely right up there, next to godliness.

Alongside a growing interest in dieting and exercising, hygiene became a sign of individual 'enlightenment' and self-discipline. 'Cleanliness' was a key component within the social identity of the British middle and upper classes – blankets, curtains, airy rooms, soap and drains were all referred to as 'English comforts'.[4]

From the 19th century until relatively recently, personal hygiene served these key purposes:

❖ A prophylactic against disease

❖ Protection from biological pathogens

❖ An integral part of moral and spiritual self-identity

❖ A status symbol in society

History Repeats Itself

Today, in the 21st century, we have such a deep applied knowledge and understanding of microbes, as well as of disease transmission, that you might imagine we're totally protected from external pathogens. And in many ways that's true. Our life expectancy has doubled and many killer diseases and epidemics are a thing of the past.

Many of us are living a lot longer and most of us also want to live *well*. I'm sure you'll agree that the prospect of living a long life *without* good health and a sense of wellbeing isn't very appealing. In fact, 'wellbeing' is such a buzzword these days – it seems everyone's talking about it. But at the same time we're witnessing an epidemic of chronic tiredness, loneliness, emotional overload and mental burnout.

Although a doctor might declare us healthy, so many of us are still trapped in a state of feeling unwell. Holistic health practices are opening up in every town, but people still can't seem to achieve *sustainable* wellness. And by that I don't mean just going through a good phase, but having wellness as a habitual, default state.

There's a reason I chose to open this book with a brief history of hygiene: comparing our earlier behaviour and attitudes with our modern-day ones can teach us how change occurs in society, and it can also help us to learn from our mistakes. But I'm afraid that previous mistakes in attitude are exactly what we're repeating when managing our wellbeing.

As we've discussed, until relatively recently people didn't really 'own' their bodies. They were at the mercy of pathogens they didn't know about, and their environment pretty much dictated their lifespan and their general quality of life, as well as the success (or otherwise) of their attempts to avoid disease. I think it's true to say that the invisible realm of germs ruled the world.

However, as I mentioned earlier, there is also a different form of contamination. It's invisible, and therefore many of us don't yet know about it: in the same way that our ancestors didn't have a clue about the biological pathogens inhabiting their bodies and their environment. I'm talking about our overexposure to toxic energies and vibrations.

The truth is that we're simply unfamiliar with our intrinsic energy and its rules of self-care, and as a result we're left open to all sorts of external forms of energy and influences. These are all around us, just like microbes, but even if you had the most powerful microscope in the world you still wouldn't be able to see them.

I hope that one day soon a scientist will invent an instrument that allows everyone to see the various forms of energy for themselves. However, for now, in common with many other energy healers, I rely on my hands to do the energy 'seeing'. My hands serve as my microscope!

Your Catalyst for Sustainable Wellness

As someone who has built a thriving practice based on long-lasting results, I believe the insights I've gained from my patients' cases are of value to those of you who have picked up this book. This is why I'm going to share my catalysts for sustainable wellness and provide you with the missing pieces of the health jigsaw puzzle – even though they're invisible – to complete your outlook on wellbeing.

In my energy healing practice, I always form a team with a patient so we can both address the issues from *all* angles; I do this because true health isn't possible without an individual taking responsibility for themselves and understanding their environment. If they fail to do this, they will resemble those patients from the dark ages of medicine who took cures for an upset stomach while simultaneously drinking dirty water.

In fact, it's of great importance that, alongside our usual personal hygiene rituals, we *all* take care of our 'energy hygiene'. It should become one of the pillars of our self-care, regardless of whether we'd like to enhance our wellbeing or form a better team with a doctor or practitioner. However, our approach to energy hygiene should go deeper than just 'masking the odour' of the imbalance in our energy, as our ancestors did with their bodily hygiene. Later in this book I'll reveal to you the real causes of energy toxicity, so you can tackle it at the root.

Another of my big passions is trying to make wellness accessible to everyone, and integrated into daily life. The media so often portrays a wellness lifestyle as a luxury, obtainable only by the well heeled. Wellness is marketed as a combination of expensive getaways, advanced yoga poses and exotic food. As a result, far too many people view a sense of wellness as a treat, rather than something that's perfectly normal.

However, once you establish a healthier and cleaner relationship with your own energy and the energy of your environment, you won't need to go to a faraway land to find your true self or to unwind. It's not about being in a particular setting but about the quality of your interaction with what surrounds you.

I think the time has come to move away from the prejudices and ignorance, which are similar to the ones our ancestors faced when dealing with the 'unseen', and to change not only our attitude towards the world of energy but also the belief that wellness routines are the preserve of the privileged few. Wellbeing isn't a status symbol, it's a necessity: just like our daily shower or bath.

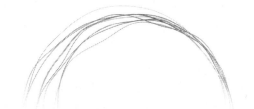

My Path to Living My Truth

'Mama, why do I have these sensations in my hand?' 'Why am I sensing things in this way?' Those are the kinds of questions I was asking as a young girl, and I'm truly blessed that my mother didn't dismiss my questions but honoured them with answers and explanations.

There's a unique reason for this: for at least the last five generations of my family all the women on my mother's side were born with the gift of healing. The older women helped the younger ones, including me, to understand their extrasensory abilities, and taught them how to utilize these to benefit other people.

However, there was a huge obstacle at the outset of my own path as a healer – the fact that I was born in the USSR during the rule of the Communist Party. You may be aware that communist ideology is based on materialism and is strictly opposed to any form of spirituality and metaphysics. The Soviet regime believed that spiritual beliefs were 'the opium of the people' and that only Marxist-Leninist doctrines could lead to a bright future and happiness.

Anyone who dared to follow a path that wasn't in sync with communist ideology, or who was interested in anything different or foreign, was viewed with suspicion – or even as an enemy of the state. The Soviet government assumed full responsibility for the Russian people's lifestyle needs but, in return, they had to serve and worship the regime and protect its ideology.

Therefore, people like my mother, who wanted to share her healing gift to help others and master herself, had to be incredibly discreet when it came to practising it. She was a chemotherapist, treating cancer patients at a clinic, but she found a way to conduct healing sessions in our Moscow apartment once her working day was over. Looking back, I think it was extremely brave of her to do this, and my heart is full of admiration for her dedication to sharing her healing in such a high-risk environment.

My Training as an Energy Healer

The fact that my mother's healing sessions took place in our home also worked to my benefit. From a very young age, I had the opportunity to watch the way she treated her patients and how she interacted with them, and I learned a great deal from this.

My mother explained to me that the human body is surrounded by an 'energy field', or aura, and she showed me how to decode its vibrational 'pulse', or 'frequency'. I became familiar with the 'wavelengths' of particular illnesses, as well as those of health. My hands learned to memorize the 'energy ID' of various medical conditions and to deal with 'blockages' in the aura. I was also coached on how to channel healing energy to harmonize the aura. (We'll be looking at these aspects of energy healing in the book).

During my healing training, my mother emphasized the importance of creating a bespoke approach to each patient's needs, and of offering them guidance for self-care that would perfectly match their unique energy ID. Even now, this is the ethos of my practice, and it's one that inspired me to write this book.

I received other powerful lessons, too. Due to the repression of the Soviet government, it was impossible at that time for healers, spiritual teachers and parapsychologists to meet in public and openly discuss healing and spiritual matters, and so some would gather in the safety and security of our kitchen. Over tea and food they would share their ideas and experiences, and exchange handwritten translations of books on healing and spirituality that had been smuggled into Moscow from abroad.

For me, it was such an honour to spend time with these people and to absorb their knowledge. It was immensely beneficial for my spiritual growth to be surrounded by those who, despite the dangerous political climate and the threat of prosecution, had found a way to live in truth, to find their 'tribe' of kindred spirits, and to share their healing with those in need. These extraordinary individuals honed my ability to cope with hostile environments and unfavourable circumstances, and to be undeterred by the opposition of sceptics. They demonstrated to me that no one can take away the freedom of our spirit – unless, of course, we allow them to do so.

The gift of healing carries with it a big responsibility for practitioners to remain pure 'channels' for energy, so it's important that we take good care of ourselves. My mother and older sister looked after their health and wellbeing by regularly fasting, meditating and eating healthy food. In fact, following a healthy lifestyle on all levels was the norm in my home and was considered a necessity rather than an indulgent luxury.

I was also incredibly fortunate that my father, a scientist with a PhD in mechanical engineering, accepted the power of healing rather than dismissing it. Dad didn't want to deny the fact of the aura or the existence of energy healing just because it didn't fit with his logical mind or with scientific principles. Throughout his life he was incredibly proud of the gifts my mother, sister and I possessed, and he loved to hear about our case studies and the successful outcomes of our energy work.

Until his final days, he attended almost all of my seminars and lectures, and was very touched by the fact that our family's healing methods were helping so many. He completely accepted what was manifesting in front of his eyes, rather than becoming blinkered by scientific knowledge, a rigid mind and a fear of going against mainstream views.

This powerful acceptance gave me a huge amount of confidence, especially when dealing with the cynicism of non-seekers. Through Dad, I came to believe that scientists should never lose their curiosity and sense of wonder while they're trying to expand our understanding of the world.

So, as you can see, my training as an energy healer and my acquisition of esoteric knowledge had to be conducted in secret: undercover, if you like. My official study of the workings of the human body, however, continued at medical school in Moscow. Believing that I'd never be able to use my healing abilities openly, I reasoned that pursuing mainstream medicine would at least allow me to stay within the healthcare profession.

Today, I'm deeply appreciative of my study of orthodox medicine, as it enables me to form a holistic view of my patients' needs. I don't regard any healing modality as 'alternative' medicine, but only as a complementary one. Both schools of medicine have the right to exist and, most importantly, to intertwine with and enhance one another.

I decided to complete my pursuit of orthodox medicine when President Gorbachev's political programme of perestroika and glasnost revolutionized Russia in the late 1980s. Life became more liberal and relaxed, and the people were allowed freedom of expression. The old Russian tradition of healing re-emerged and people turned once more to spirituality for guidance rather than to communist doctrines.

Getting Established Against All Odds

After the collapse of the Soviet Union in 1991, things changed dramatically for both my mother and me. It was as though a window had been opened and we could breathe freely at last. The air was filled with excitement at all the new opportunities and freedom. My mother left the medical clinic where she'd been working and, alongside other healer colleagues, founded one of the first healing centres in Moscow. This, of course, would have been absolutely unthinkable in communist Russia.

I'd always been drawn to the eclectic approach to holistic medicine, so I travelled to South Asia to study acupuncture and other natural therapies. In the early 1990s, my life path led me to the UK, which has been my home ever since. To my astonishment, however, when I first arrived in the country, my work was greeted by an attitude that wasn't dissimilar to that of the Communist Party!

For many, the type of healing I was practising was simply too ethereal, too inexplicable, too foreign, and way too different from the socially acceptable, mainstream forms of healing. People allowed their prejudices to hold sway, without even bothering to try it for themselves. I was met not only with scepticism – which could at least be reversed in the presence of the facts – but also by blatant cynicism.

I found that although some people were interested in the various forms of complementary medicine, energy healing was simply a step too far. So, although healing practitioners were permitted to offer their services in the UK, many of the people I met were unwilling to open their minds to something new and different. During that period I was particularly grateful to all the healers from my former life in the Soviet Union, who showed me how to stay strong and confident in the face of ridicule and opposition.

In the early days after setting up my practice, I found it was attracting a particular kind of patient: those with seemingly hopeless health problems who were prepared to try energy healing as a 'last resort'. Today, it still saddens me that many of us will open our minds and accept the non-physical, spiritual side of our nature only as a result of pain and desperation.

So, step by step, I built up my practice with these very challenging cases. And when I was able to resolve them all successfully, it served as a vivid demonstration of the power of energy healing. Slowly, word-of-mouth recommendations turned my practice into one of the most in-demand in London.

In the mid-1990s, the 'Cool Britannia' period created such a buzz in the UK. As with the years of perestroika and glasnost in the USSR, it was an incredibly exciting time. The country became more outward facing and open to new and original ideas; coming after the depression of the early 1990s' economic recession, it was a very optimistic era in which creative individuality was encouraged.

Yoga, organic food and alternative medicine became more mainstream; and people adopted more expressive and less reserved ways of being. And, once again, just as I'd done in my homeland, I was breathing in the air of change and unlimited possibilities! Leading British glossy magazines started to write about my healing practice, and I was invited to work at The Life Centre, one of the UK's first centres for yoga and healing.

My Inspiration for This Book

I've come a long way since those tentative early days as an undercover healing student in the USSR. Today, I still run the one-to-one healing practice I established in London, and prefer to work in my own low-key way. Over the past two decades the practice has developed a global following, and has repeatedly been voted one of the top healing practices in the UK. My high success rate has won the respect of orthodox medicine consultants and my patient waiting list has become increasingly lengthy.

Another passion is running energy-balancing retreats. On these, I take my patients to special and powerful locations for an intensive recharging and rebalancing programme. I also collaborate with leading international spas and act as a senior consultant for a few, helping to integrate their medical and holistic services; additionally, I create bespoke healing experiences to kick-start spa guests' wellness process.

When I became pregnant with my daughter, I took a break from my healing practice and wrote my first book, *Energy Secrets* (Hay House), which outlined my plan for holistic wellbeing. It was translated into 16 languages, which was wonderful because I'd wanted as many people as possible to benefit from my family's time-tested energy healing methods.

My current style of healing is based on the methods used by my family, along with my inherited ability to understand the 'vibrational language' of the human body, more than 20 years' experience in healing individual patients, and an in-depth knowledge of the ancient Eastern forms of traditional medicine. And, of course, my training in orthodox medicine gives me a sophisticated understanding of the workings of the human body.

My mother, sister and I still exchange case studies and the latest healing know-how over Skype; we never stop learning from each other. I love the fact that my training allows me to find the most appropriate healing methods for each patient, and that I'm not attached to only one healing protocol. I'm an advocate of teamwork between all kinds of treatment modalities, be it orthodox medicine or the various types of holistic therapy.

People often describe my approach to wellbeing as 'no-nonsense'. Thanks to my father, I guess, I offer my guidance in a proactive, pragmatic and systematic style. I also firmly believe that my patients have to participate fully in their healing process if it's to be successful. My life's lessons and challenges, and my fight for the survival of my authentic self, have convinced me that it's *essential* we own our energy, regardless of the circumstances, and protect our unique energy ID, which is why I felt compelled to write this book.

My inspiration also came from my amazing patients and their incredible success stories, and my passion for raising awareness of the vital importance of managing and owning our energy. It also came from my father, who never stopped owning his energy, even when the cancer was taking over his body. He wouldn't allow the label of his diagnosis, the grim realities of his hospital stays, intrusive medical interventions or physical pain to rob him of his authentic energy vibrations.

So, are *you* ready to start reclaiming your energy and own it as a victor? Let's get started.

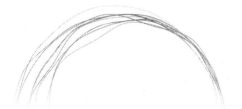

Introduction

*'If you want to find the secrets of the Universe,
think in terms of energy, frequency and vibration.'*

NIKOLA TESLA, SERBIAN-AMERICAN PHYSICIST

As a fifth-generation healer, I can confidently declare that Tesla's insight also applies to finding the secrets of our wellbeing. Despite a massive shift in our attitudes towards personal health and wellness in recent decades, many of us are still trapped in an endless cycle of imbalance-rebalance-sabotage, wondering why we never get better or feel happier, even though we seem to be doing everything we can to get well.

Many of us have problems that tend to repeat themselves, so perhaps there's something amiss with our perspective on wellness, and on the Self? Through my healing practice, I've discovered that if we work only with the physical body, when the root of the problem lies in our *energy*, the 'cure' can only be temporary and the problem will return, over and over again.

I think it's a tragedy that this widespread ignorance of the vital role that energy plays in our life and health means that so many of us are destined to have limited health, and therefore a limited life.

Getting to Know Your Driver

In his most famous equation, $E = mc^2$, Albert Einstein showed us that matter (the solids, liquids and gases all around us and out in the Universe) is a form of energy: in fact, energy and matter are essentially two side of the same coin. And you may be aware that for many thousands of years, Eastern cultures have successfully practised energy medicine, including Ayurveda and acupuncture.

Even if you've never experienced this type of healing, I'm willing to bet that you've experienced energy at work in your life. For example, have you ever responded to a situation by drawing on what you'd call your sixth sense: your intuition? Do you find that being around certain people leaves you feeling drained, while the company of others lifts your mood? Have you ever said of someone, 'There was chemistry between us'? And have you ever walked into a room and felt the energy was so heavy you could 'cut it with a knife'?

These are just some of manifestations of the energy I'm talking about, the energy that we need to recognize in ourselves in order to enhance our life and our wellbeing. Yet, here in the West, so many people are still choosing to *ignore* energy, even though it serves as a vital template for our health, our environment and our life path. They form an opinion about it based on ignorance, rather than being open-minded enough to learn exactly what it is and how it works and then make an informed judgement.

Imagine for a moment that your body is a taxi. If you want it to take you somewhere, or to do or achieve something, you have to tell the driver where to go. Now, imagine that the driver is your energy. If you talk to the car, you won't get anywhere – you need to address the driver directly. One of the reasons we keep failing to attain health or fulfilment in life (or both) is because the vast majority of us aren't talking to the right part of ourselves. We simply haven't worked out who's the boss!

Join My Dream Team

As a highly skilled and experienced energy healer, I believe that it's my duty not only to treat people but also to empower them to become masters of their own wellbeing and to harness their invisible driving life forces.

This book, along with my previous two (*Energy Secrets* and *Your Secret Laws of Power*), was inspired by the invaluable insights I've gained from the people who've attended my healing practice. One of my great professional passions is identifying and then implementing the triggers or catalysts that will help launch a patient's transformation to wellness. It's the application of these, above all, that has led to my practice's high success rate for more than 20 years.

During the healing process, I don't turn my patients into dependent disciples or passive energy recipients. Instead, I encourage each one to become my team-mate; after all, there are three of us involved: me, the patient, and the patient's problem.

I stress that it's absolutely crucial that people take full responsibility for their body and their emotions. If you choose a quick fix or just 'buy' energy, you'll be forever on a carousel of temporary improvement, or under the illusion that things are changing. You can buy something to soothe you, but you can never buy change. Instead, you have to earn it, and my intention in this book is to give you the tools and the know-how to do so.

I'm offering you my healing hands and inviting you to form a team with me. Together we'll focus on a practical application of metaphysical knowledge, and I'll reveal my breakthrough insights for achieving lasting health and vitality.

Forget Perfection, Choose Authenticity

As I explained earlier, every human has a personal energy field – known as an aura – and it's *unique* in its expression. The outline of the aura varies in diameter from person to person, so we all have a particular auric shape. Our aura isn't static, like a frozen cloud around us: instead, its *waves of energy* are constantly moving, or *vibrating*, at a *frequency* that's unique to us. These waves of energy flow through the key energy centres and channels in the aura (you'll learn about these later). The unique frequency of our aura is also our *authentic* frequency.

These parameters of the aura are so specific to each person that they almost resemble a passport, or as I call it, an *energy ID*. Just as no two fingerprints or snowflakes are alike, so we are all different in our energy ID. (Don't worry if you're still not clear on what energy and the aura are: we'll be exploring them in more depth soon).

One of the key ideas in this book is that true happiness and freedom and a meaningful existence are possible only when we lead an *authentic* life. And to do this we need to maintain and protect the unique, authentic frequency of our aura and *own* our energy.

By authentic I mean daring to be yourself – living in alignment with your own values and feeling that you're on the right path; and that, no matter what comes your way, you're able to say 'yes' to the things that resonate with you and 'no' to the things that don't. Being authentic also means respecting your personal boundaries and those of other people.

Right now, you may be asking yourself, *Why would I want to lead an authentic life? Isn't my life OK as it is?* So many of us have a deep-seated belief that living authentically is selfish, and so we spend an inordinate amount of energy trying to silence our intuition, our inner voice, in order to stay attuned to the energy of other people.

We may feel that our personal boundaries are a nuisance to others; and if we suffer from low self-esteem, we may even feel empathy for those who resist them. So, we tend to prioritize other people's feelings over what feels right for us, and we use their happiness as our point of reference. All of this leads us to *disown* our energy.

Walk Your Own Path

However, it's essential for each of us to be *in control* of our own energy. If we aren't, we're giving that control to someone or something else. When we're deficient in energy, or we undermine our personal boundaries, we're taken over by the energies of the people around us, or by the energy of our problems, and end up feeling lost in life, no longer knowing who we are. We'll be looking at these issues later in the book.

We all know that our car requires a particular type of fuel, or that our electronic devices need an appropriate charger or a particular type of battery. Our aura too must be fed with the *right kind* of energy – the energy that matches our energy ID. In this book, we'll be looking at our personal boundaries as filters that exist to protect us from the wrong type of energy consumption; without them, our aura will be damaged – just as our devices are when we use inappropriate sources or types of energy.

Your intuition, when used in combination with the exercises in this book, will help you to refine your personal 'port' so it will only allow in appropriate kinds of vibrations. You'll also figure out what your 'fuel' is and how to obtain it in a healthy, sustainable way.

When choosing to lead an authentic life you must examine your motivation and keep it in check. However, if you have a 'keeping up with the Joneses' kind of motivation, you'll never own your energy. You'll only ever be owned by the energy of other people's approval and reactions.

So many people disconnect from their authentic life force because they forget this simple truth: the energy of your free will is a lot stronger than the energy of your stars or your fate. When you refuse to give up and crumble under difficult circumstances, you're stronger than your destiny. Don't allow anything (including horoscopes, birth charts or adversaries) or anyone to write the narrative of your life story. Nothing is above your free will, which is an integral part of your unique energy ID.

I've seen many people who exist in a projected 'template', shaped by someone else's predictions or another's limitations, instead of being artisans of their own life path. Throughout this book, I'll be showing you how to own your energy and your unique energy frequency, so that you can be your true self, walk your own path and create a unique legacy. In this way, owning your energy will become an integral part of leading an authentic life.

Energy Exchange Between People

Another of the book's central themes is a potentially life-changing insight that came to me after years of hands-on practice and from studying my healing family's cases. My breakthrough realization is that we are naturally and continually attuning to each other's energy, and moreover have a tendency to synchronize our auric waves with others' auras. Until recently, it was believed that this tendency was reserved only for empaths or highly sensitive people.

Many of you may already have noticed that you try to synchronize your steps, the tone of your voice and your body language when interacting with others. You'll have experienced too the effects of a 'contagious laugh' and the feeling of being 'brought down' by the mere presence of a particular person.

Some of you may have used the ancient art of feng shui, which encourages a sense of wellbeing by harmonizing our energy with the energy of our environment. For thousands of years, billions of people throughout Asia treated this knowledge with the utmost respect, due to its profound effects on both wellness and life in general.

Later, we'll be looking in greater detail at the scientific research relating to such *synchronicity* between living organisms and the ways in which our environment affects us biologically and physiologically.

We are all 'one' – connected by the invisible exchange network of human energy. But this doesn't mean we have to lose our authenticity or stop being autonomous. I will be revealing to you the secrets behind your ability to 'catch' energy and showing you how to master it. You'll also learn how to become discerning with your natural ability to synchronize with other people.

A Clean Aura = Sustainable Wellness

Another of the principal concepts in this book is that we sabotage our state of balance by failing to ensure that our aura remains true to its authentic energy ID. There are multiple reasons why we do this and we'll be looking at every one of them, but the bottom line is that as well as taking care of our physical body, we also need to look after our aura.

We often confuse being 'open' with other people with the entirely different matter of 'energetic promiscuity'. Let me explain what I mean by this before you get the wrong idea! I'm pretty sure you wouldn't allow anyone and everyone to put their hands under your clothes – that would be nothing less than abuse – and that you exercise careful judgement before seeking intimacy with another person. However, many of us allow absolutely *everything* to get 'under our skin' at an energetic level, which means we don't exercise the same discretion with our energy as we do with our physical body.

Many people are unaware that being 'open' is not the same as discarding the concept of being discerning with our energy and protecting our personal boundaries. This misunderstanding has allowed too many energies to crash through our (nonexistent) boundaries and overexpose the sacred parts of our being to a negative influence, or something that's abusive. A big clue that this has happened comes when we can't get negative people out of our system, or we turn ourselves into a 'rubbish bin' so the people around us can unload their bad day onto us, and we just soak it up.

Interestingly, the vibrations of other people's energy (you'll learn about these later) can infiltrate our aura in a similar way to the biological pathogens that penetrate our physical body. Others' dominant energy can 'reprogramme' us or even crash our system, just like a virus invading the nucleus of our cells. Even if our aura isn't compromised in this way, it may instead be contaminated with 'toxic energy', just as the body is exposed to bacteria. What's more, our natural defence mechanism is incredibly similar in principle to our immune system. I'll explain these fascinating links, and more, later in the book.

Just as your everyday personal hygiene methods are designed to keep you clean and prevent you from hosting and spreading germs, the 'energy hygiene' I'll be teaching you focuses on keeping your aura in a pure and authentic state, and it will protect you from anything that can sabotage your energy ID.

A clean aura brings physical, mental and emotional wellbeing: it allows for new energy to come into your life. Only then can you manifest the miracle of profound change and literally become 'attractive' – pulling positive vibrations into your orbit. It's only when your aura is clean that you can own your energy. Otherwise, you'll be owned by the energy of others and become sidetracked from your unique path, forever wondering when you'll begin to live your own life!

Many people only start looking into energy clearing as a result of contracting a disease, but I'll be encouraging *you* to incorporate energy hygiene into your daily routine right away, and make it an integral part of a healthy lifestyle.

Doing What Works

I'm a hands-on practitioner from a long line of healers, and I treat people every day, so all my techniques are tested, tried and perfected for maximum impact. The meditations, visualizations and other tools I've shared in this book are designed to take you to the threshold of infinite possibilities so you can reclaim your unique energy ID and life path. I know what works and what's less effective.

Please practise the exercises in this book with an open mind. In fact, if you find yourself baulking at a particular one or thinking, *There's no way I'm going to do that!* consider carefully why you're reacting in that way. We often shy away from the things we need the most, so it could well be that this is *precisely* the exercise that can help you.

Change starts at the edge of our comfort zone. This means you won't shift while you're attached to what you already know. Of course, many people exist in a comfortably numb state or in stagnation, but that's not what it means to be alive!

Please try to step out of familiar territory and allow yourself a fresh perspective. I realize this is a challenging concept, and that it can take courage to see it through. You may even be telling yourself that you're perfectly happy just as you are. However, even if you're not yet ready to embrace the idea of transformation – something I encourage in my patients – you might at least agree that there's always scope for enhancing the life you have now. Things can always be a little bit better!

You must be willing for this to happen to you if you want my tools to work for you. If you'd prefer to stay exactly as you are at the moment, you won't experience the range of benefits that this book has the power to offer you. Some of my techniques may not feel entirely comfortable at first, but if you're willing to explore them they will help you to grow. Think of it as like joining a gym. You may only go when you trust that it will benefit you, and it may take a lot of effort and willpower at first, but once you start, you soon begin to feel good, and when you see and experience the results you're happy to keep going.

Throughout this book, I'm going to ask you questions that are designed to shake you out of your comfort zone, so you can find and reclaim your unique energy ID. This will reset your system, rather than simply patch it up. Just as we occasionally need to reinstall the software on our computer, as you work with each chapter, you'll be rebooting your energy system, rather than just repairing it. With the help of my healing methods, you'll be dissecting your life, layer by layer, to check for any possible contamination in your aura, reflect on the diet of your life's choices, and analyse your social and living environments.

I recognize that I'm expecting a lot from you as you work with this book. There's a great deal of information for you to absorb, so I advise you to start at the beginning and work carefully through to the end. I do appreciate that many of you are busy people living in the real world, so I've adapted my recommendations and techniques to fit everyday reality.

As I say, some of my insights may challenge your perceptions; however, although you may not sense energy in the same way that I do, you're still affected by it all the time, every day. Your energy is invisible, but that's not to say it doesn't exist!

At present, you may be unaware of the effects of failing to protect your energy and leading an inauthentic life, although you may be experiencing them nonetheless. Not long ago we were unaware of the damaging effects of UV rays and, as a result, spent years sunbathing without applying SPF cream. We couldn't grasp the fact that too much sun exposure is harmful, but today we know it can lead to skin cancer.

I've written this book to inform you of other types of invisible emissions – auric ones. These too have the potential to damage your life, yet they can also bring so much goodness and empower you with insights into what will keep you protected from harmful energy. However, this book isn't only about protection – just as importantly, it will show you how to be discerning with your energy.

Perhaps one day scientists will confirm my theories about the effects that others' energy can have on us. In the meantime, I hope this book will help you to lead a much more authentic and energetic life.

Today, we are experiencing an epidemic of mutual energy abuse, and generic living is becoming the norm. This is leading to the destruction of the Self and of our planet, too, because inauthenticity disconnects us from the instinct of self-preservation. *Energy Rules* is my call for you to reveal your authentic energy ID, so the world will gain a shining soul and you'll feel truly alive in the uniqueness of your energy expression.

Part I

ENERGY:
BEYOND
THE
VISIBLE
DIMENSION

CHAPTER 1

Unlocking the Mystery of You

At its most basic level, your body – and in fact, all life, as well as the non-living world – is made up of tiny units called atoms. Quantum physics – the branch of science that describes nature at its smallest scale of atoms and subatomic particles – tells us that atoms are not solid and that as we go deeper and deeper into their structure we see that they consist mostly of empty space.

In fact, the atom is actually a force field, like a miniature tornado, which emits waves of *energy*. This means that everything in the Universe is made up of energy, rather than matter, even when it appears to be completely inert and solid. Atoms, and therefore everything else in the Universe, are also *vibrating* at a particular *frequency*; we'll be looking at this in more depth later.

We live in a 'soup' of all kinds of energy waves, and we ourselves are *energy beings*. The book or ebook reader you're holding might look static and solid, but quantum physics has taught us that it's anything but: it's teeming with subatomic particles that are in a perpetual state of motion. The table I'm sitting at as I write these words looks solid, and I'll certainly realize how hard it is if I bang my knee against it when I get up from my chair, but it too is composed of subatomic particles that are whizzing around at superfast speed.

Like all light and matter, these subatomic particles behave in two different ways simultaneously. In what's known as wave-particle duality, subatomic particles exhibit the properties of both particles *and* waves. So therefore, we, like everything else in the Universe, are 100 per cent wave and 100 per cent particle.

In the West, the popular perception of the body is that it consists of solid matter. However, quantum physicists, Eastern masters, and healers such as myself accept that our bodies are made up of energy. Please don't worry if you're struggling to get your head around this! I haven't written this book to explain the complexities of quantum physics, though, and you certainly don't need to know anything more about it to benefit from what I'm about to teach you. *Energy Rules* is about the practical application of metaphysical knowledge to enhance our wellness.

Introducing Your Aura

The idea that you're an energy being might be a tough one to accept, but it's truly essential that you do; and I'm sure you'll find it very beneficial once you get used to it. I'm going to adopt some of the principles of Eastern philosophy as I teach you about your energy essence in this chapter, as they are very clear and all encompassing.

As we discussed in the Introduction, every one of us has an invisible energy field, or aura, that extends around our body. Our aura doesn't exist independently from nature: it's brought into being when two opposing primal magnetic forces collide in our physical body. One force travels up from the ground (terrestrial) while the other bears down on us from above (Universal).

Although illustrations of the aura often make it look like a shell that surrounds us and is separate from us, that isn't the case. In fact, we're soaked in our aura, just as a foetus in the womb is soaked in amniotic fluid.

As you learned earlier, your aura has certain parameters that form your unique energy ID. The shape of your aura is different to mine and everyone else's and its waves of energy are vibrating at a frequency that's unique to you.

In fact, it's true to say that you, like everyone else, are simply a unique 'wave' of energy. Sometimes you'll encounter people with a similar vibrational frequency to your own, and remark that you're 'on the same wavelength' as them. You might think that's just a figure of speech but you're actually describing the nature of your affinity with that person.

I would also like to highlight that in this book, I'm focusing on the aspects of the aura that relate to our ego self and our personal space. The soul is also part of the aura (it's the furthest-out layer) and of course it's limitless in its parameters. But that's a topic for another book!

Your aura might not yet be perceptible to you – later, I'll teach you how to engage with it – but it is to me, and to other healers. As an energy healer, I work with the human aura on a daily basis. My extrasensory gift enables me to 'read' a patient's aura and retune it so it has what I call an authentic balance (we'll talk more about this later).

DETECT YOUR AURA

You might like to try this simple exercise to sense your auric energy, so you're not only connecting to the information in this chapter cerebrally but viscerally, too.

✧ Rub your hands together, briskly and vigorously, for around 10–15 seconds.

✧ Now pull your hands away from each other until they are about 10–15 cm (4–6 inches) apart, and keep them there. At this point, many people sense that their hands are 'holding' a ball full of a magnetic force, and they are surprised at how palpable it feels.

✧ You can intensify this sensation by moving your hands slightly towards and away from each other.

✧ What is it you're feeling? It's your aura!

The Form and Function of the Aura

The aura is made up of seven layers, or currents, of energy, each of which has a unique purpose and quality. Some people compare the structure of the aura with the layers of an onion, but as a Russian I prefer to draw a comparison with the famous Russian doll *matryoshka*. Our physical body is the smallest doll and around that are the other seven layers of our aura, each larger than the previous one.

However, unlike the *matryoshka*, each layer or energy current is interrelated, and each one affects the others. They also affect our

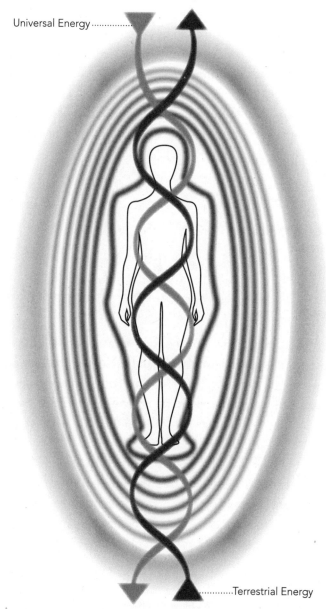

Universal Energy

Terrestrial Energy

Image 1 – The aura and the direction of primal energy forces
(Note: crossover points are not precise and are for general guidance only)

7

feelings, emotions, thought patterns, behaviour and overall health and wellbeing. In this book, I'm going to focus on the three layers of the aura that are closest to the physical body. If you'd like to familiarize yourself with the other layers of the aura, you can read my book *Energy Secrets*.

These are the three layers of the aura you'll be working on when you do the exercises and meditations coming up later in the book:

1. The physical layer

2. The emotional layer

3. The mental layer

Let's take a look at each of these in turn:

The Physical Layer

This is the densest layer of the aura because it's the one that's closest to your physical body. If you could see this layer, you'd realize that it's an exact copy of your body: each organ, each structure, has its counterpart here. It permeates right through your physical body, following its contours, and usually extends beyond it by 3–5 cm (1–2 inches).

The physical layer of the aura is also known as the energy matrix, because it forms the bridge between the physical world around us and the non-physical states of energy. The physical layer is covered in energetic channels, also known as meridians, which link specific areas of the body with each other. We'll explore the meridians shortly.

Acupuncturists and practitioners of traditional Chinese medicine, in particular, work very closely with the meridians, but other healing disciplines use them too. Any changes in your organs or physiology are reflected in the state of the physical layer, so it serves as an invaluable indicator of your overall physical health.

The Emotional Layer

The second layer of the aura reflects our emotional history and our current emotional state. It's clearly defined in shape and extends outside the physical body by roughly 5–10 cm (2–4 inches). However, the size of this layer really depends on our emotional intelligence – the more of that we have, the bigger this layer is.

Although its outer edges are sharply defined, the interior of this layer is always in motion. Clusters of energy matter are continually moving towards each other and then separating again, rather like a lava lamp. When you're experiencing healthy emotions, these shifting patterns of energy are smooth and free flowing, and light in colour.

However, when you're caught in the grip of negative emotions, such as jealousy, fear or anger, they become stagnant, dark and clotted. This can also have a negative impact on your physical health because the physical and emotional layers of the aura are interlinked.

When you meet someone and have an instinctive response to them – whether it's wanting to get to know them better or preferring to put as much distance between you and them as possible – it's because you're reacting to the emotional layer of their aura. We tend to connect and form empathy with people whose emotional energy is in harmony with our own. Conversely, we tend to avoid people whose emotional layer is 'blocked', due to their anger or negative moods, which weighs us down or 'shuts down' our heart.

We can also block and pollute our emotional layer if we engage in negative self-talk or negative thoughts. Which leads us to the next layer...

The Mental Layer

This is the energy of our thoughts, knowledge and experiences, and just like the other layers it's identical to the shape of our physical body. It extends roughly 10–20 cm (4–8 inches) beyond the body and flows from the top of the head downwards.

This layer can become stagnant due to our mental blocks, overly rigid opinions and narrow-mindedness, or by other people's manipulative behaviour. Entrenched and traumatic memories can also form energy blockages here, and we find that we're unable to shake off the echo of these past experiences.

The health of our mental layer is determined by our attitude to the past, and whether we're able to work through difficult experiences and release them or tend to hold on to them and replay them in our mind like a broken record. Every past event, regardless of our level of recollection, is logged in this layer, and its grip depends on our attitude towards the past and our commitment to the energy of the present moment.

The condition of our mental layer is also determined by how open-minded we are; whether we're receptive to new ideas and experiences, or instead have erected a mental wall between ourselves and theories, opinions or events that sit beyond our comfort zone. Often, blocks at this level will make us immune to change because change only happens when we're out of our comfort zone.

There is a strong link between this layer and the emotional and physical ones. Our thoughts and beliefs will always trigger an emotional response and also affect many functions and the neurological wiring of our body.

The Aura's Energy Centres and Channels

The best way to engage with our aura is through its key energy centres, known in traditional Eastern teaching as chakras, and its energy channels, also known as meridians, because these penetrate all of its layers. (This might feel like a lot of theory to grasp, but it's absolutely vital knowledge if you want to thrive in life!)

Nature has given us these powerful tools for mastering our health and life in general but, once again, because they are invisible, many of us don't know how to recognize and utilize them. We'll be using chakras and meridians throughout the book, as 'tuning keys' to balance and reclaim your energy field, or aura, and I'll show you exactly what to do.

Even just being aware of your chakras and meridians can move you towards a better balance in life, because they act as powerful allies for self-reflection. You might find that this chapter will immediately inspire you to get reacquainted with yourself at a different and more profound level than ever before.

Later, I'll be giving you vivid meditations and other exercises that will encompass all your senses, so you can utilize the power of visualization – which is one of the best ways to connect with your chakras.

The Chakras

As you now know, the aura is the result of the interaction of two force fields – the Universal (coming down) and the terrestrial (rising up). These forces cross as they travel through our body and their central crossing points are where we find the chakras. (The chakras don't have a physical form and no conventional X-ray or MRI scan can reveal their presence and location).

The chakras are whirling vortexes of energy (the word *chakra* means wheel in the ancient Indian language of Sanskrit, but to my mind they are more like tornadoes; in Eastern traditions, the chakras are often depicted as the lotus – the flower of spiritual awakening). In fact, you can think of the chakras as energy *depots* because they store the energy from the two aura-forming forces (the Universal and the terrestrial) as well as the energy from our environment and our lifestyle (diet, breathing and so on). The chakras are also responsible for transforming stored energy for our use and for the benefit of the world around us.

There are seven major chakras, almost all of which are located along the spine:

1. Base chakra

2. Navel chakra

3. Solar plexus chakra

4. Heart chakra

5. Throat chakra

6. Third eye chakra

7. Crown chakra

These highly charged energy centres in our aura spin in a clockwise direction as they move the energy of our body out into the energy field around us; and they spin counterclockwise to pull energy from our external world, our environment, into our body.

The seven chakras govern particular organs and physiological processes in our physical body, to which they send stored energy. As a result, when one of our chakras is damaged, suffering can be immediately detected in a related organ/body system in our physical body.

Each chakra adapts the passing flow of the aura's energy to its unique vibrational frequency; this frequency correlates with a colour (which as we know from school, is actually a wavelength of active, moving energy) and various sounds (in other words, vibrations of the various frequencies).

And the chakras respond to certain scents and tastes, too. As you read the description of each chakra in the chakra system section that follows, try to bring your awareness to its location in your body, and also 'taste', 'hear', 'smell' and 'see' it. Each of these energy centres encompasses the physical, emotional and mental energy of your aura, so I've explained the organs, emotions and thoughts/beliefs that resonate with each one.

The Chakras' Dual Expression

What I'm about to share with you is crucial, but frequently overlooked, information about the chakras. The navel, solar plexus, heart, throat and third eye chakras have two energy vortexes: one at the back and another at the front. You can imagine each of these chakras as a horizontal sand clock with your body positioned in the middle of it.

In these chakras, the purpose of the rear vortex is to accumulate energy, so you can see this as your energy bank, or your potential. The front vortex is programmed to probe external energies and, importantly, to radiate the energy and characteristics of each chakra into the world.

The base and crown chakras are different because they possess single, funnel-like energy vortexes; however, these are just as powerful as those of the dual chakras, if not more so. The base chakra opens towards the ground to connect with terrestrial energy and the crown opens towards the sky, connecting with the Universe. Nevertheless, in addition to drawing in energy, these two chakras must also spin to channel energy outwards, to share with the world.

Today, there are many people whose mindset is entirely consumerist, and even when they are working with the chakras their focus is on accumulating energy in order to elevate their own spirit. You can do all sorts of meditation, yoga and energy practices, but if your chakras are not channelling energy *outwards*, to benefit the environment, other people and the society in which you live, your aura will never be healthy.

For example, I've met a number of people who practise loving kindness meditations at a yoga centre but then make unkind remarks or engage in vicious gossip in the changing area after the class. I also know people who are interested only in spiritual topics, considering earthly issues almost beyond their concern. Yet our souls need earthly experiences as well as spiritual ones. We have to be anchored in the world. After all, we're part of it!

The higher and wider the branches of a tree grow, the deeper and wider its roots extend, and it's the same with us. The more we express the spiritual aspects of ourselves and engage with our aura, the more we're able to and must invest in anchoring and engagement in our physical, human, earthly life. Just as there's no lotus flower without the mud it grows in, there's no chance of awakening our energy without 'muddy' life experiences. So, in my opinion, dwelling solely in the spiritual realms is unlikely to create a holistic shift in a person's aura.

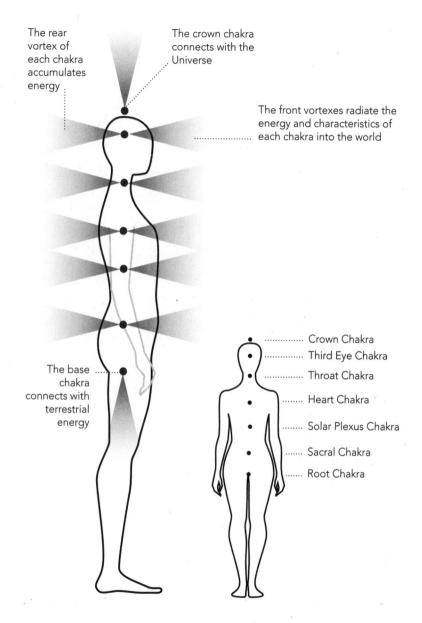

The rear vortex of each chakra accumulates energy

The crown chakra connects with the Universe

The front vortexes radiate the energy and characteristics of each chakra into the world

The base chakra connects with terrestrial energy

.... Crown Chakra
.... Third Eye Chakra
.... Throat Chakra
.... Heart Chakra
.... Solar Plexus Chakra
.... Sacral Chakra
.... Root Chakra

The Chakras' Dual Expression

The Chakra System

Our chakras must perform their purpose in the material world, as I describe below, or they will become blocked, or out of balance, and unable to spin correctly, and our energy flow will also be blocked. In time, this blockage can lead to physical symptoms in the associated organs/body systems, affect our psycho-emotional state, and sabotage our life's path and intentions. So, knowing about and caring for your chakras will have a positive, holistic effect on your health and your life in general.

The following is a very brief journey through the chakra system that will provide you with the key information you need in order to work with this book.

Base Chakra

Physical location: between the genitals and the anus

Colour: ruby red

Musical note: doh (C)

Sound: bongo drums

Scent: cinnamon, freshly cut grass, wet rock, earth

Element: earth

Taste: cherries, tomatoes, red peppers, home-cooked food

Organs/body systems: uterus, prostate, anus, legs, large bowel, sacrum

Belief: 'I am safe'

Inward expression: connection to the Earth and absorption of terrestrial energy; ability to survive; confidence; stability; grounding; letting go

Outward expression: paying household bills on time; tidiness; keeping order in all affairs associated with your survival; making peace with family members; creating a home; getting to know your neighbours; establishing a healthy routine; gardening; looking after your body.

Navel Chakra

Physical location: between the pubic area and the navel

Colour: orange-gold

Musical note: ray (D)

Sound: ocean/sea waves, waterfall

Scent: your favourite scent; orange blossom; the smell of a baby's skin; vanilla; jasmine

Element: water

Taste: carrots; satsumas; sweet potatoes; exotic food; special treats

Organs/body systems: immune system; adrenal glands; kidneys; bladder; ovaries; lumbar spine

Belief: 'I deserve'

Inward expression: absorbs and stores energy from our diet; sexuality; sensuality; pleasure; joy; playfulness; creativity

Outward expression: honour; your sensual needs; learning to nourish your senses by connecting to aromas, textures, tastes and sensations that you like and enjoy; dancing; learning to receive; improving your diet.

Solar Plexus Chakra

Physical location: solar plexus

Colour: yellow-gold

Musical note: me (E)

Sound: a roaring fire

Scent: lemon; freshly baked bread and pastry

Element: fire

Taste: bananas; yellow peppers; melon; corn; buckwheat; whole grains; sprouted seeds

Organs/body systems: stomach; liver; pancreas; spleen; small intestines; thoracic spine; lower respiratory system

Belief: 'I am powerful'

Inward expression: protection from the hostile environment; vitality; personal magnetism and charisma; zest for life; proactivity; willpower; authentic choices; commitment to choices; connection to social circles/friends

Outward expression: learning to take a calculated risk and push yourself out of your comfort zone; writing a mission statement for your life; learning to respect other people's choices; creating boundaries for yourself and honouring the boundaries of others; supporting others; admiring people's achievements; learning to let go of jealousy; creating a proactive plan to achieve your goals; reading books by people whose life story inspires you and ignites your personal power; creating a much better life/work balance; seeking career advice if not fulfilled at work.

Heart Chakra

Physical location: centre of the chest, equidistant between your nipples

Colour: grass-green

Musical note: fah (F)

Sound: wind

Scent: rose

Element: air

Taste: broccoli; courgettes; green apples; spinach; lettuce; kiwi fruit

Organs/body systems: heart; cardiovascular system; biorhythms; lower respiratory system; shoulders; lower trapezius muscles

Belief: 'I am love'

Inward expression: emotional centre; ability to accept love and love others unconditionally; self-love; compassion; kindness

Outward expression: forgiveness of others and yourself; volunteering; acts of compassion towards people around you; being more expressively romantic; having more genuine heart-to-heart connections with friends and loved ones; accepting that all people are different and deserving of compassionate acceptance; creating a daily routine that's in sync with your body's natural rhythms.

Throat Chakra

Physical location: on the neck, between the collarbone and larynx

Colour: turquoise

Musical note: soh (G)

Sound: crickets

Scent: mint; eucalyptus

Element: ether

Taste: mint; spearmint; herbal teas; aubergines; blueberries; blue corn

Organs/body systems: thyroid; cervical vertebrae; throat; upper respiratory system; lower jaw; trachea

Belief: 'I am truth'

Inward expression: honest communication; guilt resolution; clear expression; fairness; speaking the truth in balanced ways; appreciation of high forms of beauty and art; exhilaration and uplifting feelings

Outward expression: public speaking; singing; chanting; joining a local activist group whose aims resonate with you; encouraging others to express their truth; learning to listen to others, even if their point of view is different from yours; writing letters/talking to people to resolve an argument; learning not to hold your breath while listening to others; learning to silence negative inner chatter; not responding to manipulation; frequently visiting places of high art; performing daily affirmations.

Third Eye Chakra

Physical location: middle of the forehead, in the spot between your eyebrows and just above the bridge of the nose

Colour: indigo blue

Musical note: la (A)

Sound: bells

Scent: lavender; or a scent you associate with wonder/travel

Element: light

Taste: fasting

Organs/body systems: nose; ears; eyes; brain, especially the pituitary gland

Belief: 'I trust my intuition'

Inward expression: intuition; wisdom; ability to create successful tactics; effective resolution of problems; lateral thinking; imagination; visualization; focus; sharpness of perception; a flexible and open mind; freedom from conditioning; original ideas; dreams; subconscious mind; metaphysical reality

Outward expression: intuition; blocking toxins from your diet; starting to live mindfully so you can connect with life in a holistic and all-encompassing way; letting go of living on autopilot; having technology-free time every day; learning to transform your reactive attitude into a more balanced state; learning to recognize your life's lessons; allowing yourself and others to live according to the compass of personal intuition.

Crown Chakra

Physical location: just above the top of your head

Colour: white, violet

Musical note: te (B)

Sound: organ music

Scent: burning beeswax candles; myrrh; frankincense

Element: all elements in the Universe

Taste: fasting

Organs/body systems: hypothalamus; central nervous system

Belief: 'I am that I am'

Inward expression: connection to the higher Self, the Universe and the realm of spirits; enlightenment; inspiration; your intellect; your life purpose; spirituality; unity with nature; feeling at one with the soul

Outward expression: leading a drug-free life; practising daily gratitude; connecting with nature; meditation; super-conscious living serving the human Self while honouring the spirit; recognizing the cause and effect of our actions; taking responsibility for ourselves and the world around us; inspiring light in others; controlling our ego.

The Meridians

We can only feel free and truly alive when we're connected to the energy of *now*. Sadly, so many of us are feeling trapped in the past or are caught up in fantasies about the future. As a result we don't really *own* our energy – instead, it's owned by the timeline we've created for ourselves. However, it is time that should serve our life energy, not the other way round. We're only able to live consciously, taking responsibility for ourselves and those around us, when we're anchored in the present.

So, let's redress the balance and become masters of the moment.

One of the key principles for owning our life force is balancing the energies of the past, present and future. Our best allies in achieving this are the three main energy channels within the aura, through which energy flows: the meridians. In Sanskrit, their names are Ida, Pingala and Sushumna.

Just like the chakras, the meridians are invisible; and in fact, the chakras are located along the flow of the meridians. Let's have a brief look at each meridian in turn.

Ida

This is the channel of the *past*. It runs upwards and along the left side of the spine before intersecting with the third eye. Ida energy is associated with feminine energy, joy, emotions and maternal impulses. It has a strong connection with the Moon, which is why in some traditions it's known as the Moon meridian.

Ida is dominant in people who live in the past – who are caught up in nostalgia and procrastination and love to reminisce about how much better things used to be. As I mentioned, joy is connected with this meridian, so it may be that people who yearn so strongly for the past are longing to return to what they consider were happier days, and in the process they become desensitized to the joy and lightness of the present moment.

If your moods swing quickly from exhilaration and excitement to downcast and gloomy, and then back again; if you struggle to stay motivated because everything seems to require too much effort; or if you're caught up in a deep longing for the past, you may have a problem with your Ida meridian.

Pingala

This is the meridian of the *future*. It runs upwards and along the right side of the spine, through the third eye chakra and over to the left side of the brain. Pingala is also known as the Sun channel, and it's associated with masculine energy, action and planning. It's dominant in people who are living in the future: those who tell themselves that one day they'll do all sorts of things they believe they can't do right now. They are literally wishing their life away. Theirs is a 'one day it will happen' mentality.

Therefore, with its emphasis on the future, this meridian is connected with planning ahead. However, too much planning, and therefore too much emphasis on Pingala, can deplete Ida. At this point, our joy in life starts to fade and in its place comes irritation and a sense of dissatisfaction. We become annoyed with other people and may start to lose our temper over the tiniest glitch.

Sushumna

This is the meridian of the present (now), and it runs upwards in a straight line along the spinal cord, up through the third eye and crown chakras. This is your middle meridian: the channel of balance and integration.

Sushumna creates a space where our intuition can be heard, which is another important reason to strengthen this meridian. Our intuition is our best compass if we want to stay true to our life path. In fact, it's only when this meridian is dominant that you can become a 'creator' – a state that's essential for mastering your own energy and owning your life force.

Sushumna flow also awakens our soul and carries us towards spiritual evolution. It helps to balance the emotions of Ida with the actions of Pingala: our male and female sides; our ego and divine Self. The famous yogic alternate-nostril breathing technique was created to activate Sushumna and to balance all three meridians.

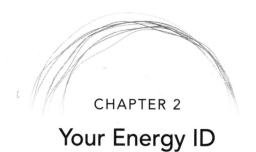

CHAPTER 2

Your Energy ID

As I explained earlier, I believe that one of the big reasons for the current wellness deficit, which is reaching epidemic proportions, is that many people don't understand the energetic component of their bodies. They think that what they see – the flesh-and-blood part of them – is all there is. They don't realize that their physical body is simply the denser, visible part of a much larger energy body – the aura.

As you're now aware, in my view this blinkered way of looking at the body leads to limited outcomes in terms of health and wellness. Our aura is a living template of our physical body, mind, emotions and our life in general. So, when it comes to trying to improve the wellness of our being, we can't just focus on the physical aspect of the Self in isolation. As I often say, the aura is the boss! In this chapter we're going to look at what makes your aura *authentic* and forms your unique energy ID.

Becoming Your Authentic Self

At this point, it's important to understand that it's only when you start to acknowledge *all* parts of yourself that you can begin to unify your power into your authentic self. As we discussed earlier, everything around us – seen and unseen – is, in its essence, a wave of energy. This energy has a vibrational frequency that's unique unto itself, and the same is true of your aura. You can only thrive in life if you find and maintain your aura's authentic frequency, otherwise you won't feel that you're resonating with your own life.

Lack of authenticity is one of the most common causes of energy loss, wellness sabotage and unhappiness. Therefore, one of the pillars of energy hygiene, which we began to discuss earlier, is the lifelong practice of authenticity. If you're not aligned with the genuine flow of your own energy, you'll simply become a magnet for all kinds of other energies, some of them harmful, and your aura will become overwhelmed by the sea of energy vibrations that surrounds you.

This will lead to auric 'clutter' that can block your vitality and cause you to attract the wrong type of people, to make choices to please others, and to feel invisible and dull. Some of my patients have described this as being 'like a cork in the sea' – continually feeling powerless, and being tossed and turned in all directions by life.

It's certainly the case that leading an authentic life might be more difficult, as it requires us to take personal responsibility; however, we can only be in the state of a 'creator' – liberated and happy – when we're being ourselves. Besides, your authentic aura will always be superior to the aura you'll have if you're copying someone else, or when you 'bend' your energy flow to please others. As Oscar Wilde said, with his customary wit, 'Be yourself, everyone else is already taken.' It's always a treat for me as a healer to come across authentic auras because they possess the most beautiful glow!

The great news is that we've *all* been created to shine, and I will help you to 'come home' to the real, genuine *you*.

Reclaiming Your Energy ID

One of the most important lessons I'll be teaching you is how to become your authentic self and how to look after it. I'll be explaining this in detail throughout the book, but it's important to introduce you to this idea now. Here are some guidelines.

1. Stay true to your unique energy ID.

2. Match your life and environment, social life and commitments to your energy frequency.

Once you've 'reclaimed your wave' it will serve as your lifelong inner point of reference and your template for creating an authentic life that resonates with your true self. You'll be able to align all the layers of your aura – in particular, your physical, emotional and mental layers – with your unique frequency. So, the *truth* will echo through your entire being.

Your Personal Space

We commonly think of personal space as a physical or psychological distance between people in a social, family or work environment, and this is largely true. However, now that you're aware of your aura you'll realize that your personal space isn't confined within the boundary of your physical body but extends a good arm's length around you.

For your aura to function properly, its energy must flow freely and expand outwards. In another words, your aura must have 'breathing space'. Your personal space is also a buffer between your inner energy system and the swirl of energies in your environment. It can be viewed as a filter that enables you to interact with those energies, while allowing through only what's beneficial for your aura and is of service to your higher good.

I'm sure that, at times, many of you have craved your personal space almost at a visceral level! You might have thought you just needed some headspace, but in reality your aura was simply suffocating under the burden of unprocessed energies. For many of us, the pace of life has speeded up dramatically, and there are increasing demands on us. We simply don't have the time or the right tools to process everything that life projects at us, including work, relationships and personal issues, and as a result, we tend to feel comfortable only when we share our personal space with people who are on the same wavelength as us. It feels good to get close and intimate with them.

The problem starts when we don't yet know our unique frequency, and therefore tend to attract random people whose presence in our energy field feels like an overwhelming intrusion. When this happens we might even describe ourselves as a sponge that soaks up everything around us.

Looking after your personal space is paramount for sustaining your wellness. Neglecting it will sabotage, over and over again, any wellness cures that you embark on. Each of us must learn how to honour and respect our personal space, because if it becomes stagnant or is nonexistent, it will become a breeding ground for energy 'pathogens' that will have a toxic effect on our life; we'll be looking at these later.

Throughout this book I'll be showing you some highly effective tools for cleaning and recovering your personal space. Once it's restored it will act as your strongest default protector against negative influences and energy overloads.

Cultural Differences

Although we all need this energetic 'breathing space', it's important to remember that every country and culture in the world sees it in a different way. Behaviour that you regard as an invasion of your personal space might be perfectly normal for someone from another culture.

For instance, people in Hispanic and Southern European countries are likely to stand in closer proximity to each other than those in Northern Europe and the United States. Russia is another country where people are happy to be close together.

So, before you assume that someone's intruding into your personal space, consider their cultural background – it could well be that the close physical proximity you're struggling with is completely acceptable in their eyes. Equally, if someone tells you to back off, it might be because their cultural background means they're used to having a lot more personal space than you are. And if someone finds you distant, it might be down to the way you were brought up. We're all different.

Your Wellness Essentials

As you've probably realized by now, true wellness can only be achieved if your approach addresses both the physical *and* the energetic aspects of your being. The two are entwined, and together they create a unity that cannot be broken.

In fact, what I've come to understand after years of practice is that you need to go one step further: you must *own* your energy. By this I mean taking responsibility for your aura and using it as your template for life. You need to adopt a self-care regimen built around the following pillars:

❖ Preventing the loss of your energy

❖ Maintaining your unique frequency

❖ Securing your personal space

Our collective failure to realize the importance of these is the main reason there's a crisis of wellness in the modern world. As I explained earlier, our ignorance of the invisible world of different energies that surrounds us, and applying a consumer mindset to our wellbeing is trapping us in the cycle of wellness-sabotage-suffering-attempted cure.

Our state of inner harmony is a fragile thing, and it's very much affected by internal and external influences. In the next part of the book I'll help you to identify what these influences might be, so you can learn how to control and master them. I'll also explain how you can achieve harmony with your environment, your family, friends and home.

My intention for those of you reading this book is the same as for my patients: I want to introduce you to another level of wellbeing that you might not even believe is possible. One in which a nourished aura, being your authentic self, and securing your personal space will forever be your pillars of a happy and healthy life.

Part II

. . . .

HUMAN ENERGY EXCHANGE: SCIENCE
AND
SURPRISES

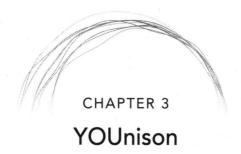

CHAPTER 3

YOUnison

Now that you're familiar with the basics of the energy concepts at the heart of this book, I'm ready to share with you the very exciting and potentially life-changing insight that came to me after many years of practice as an energy healer. Simply being aware of what I'm about to tell you can create a massive shift in your life.

There's a common belief that a person must be empathetic, or consciously willing, in order to tune in to another's state of being. And a lot has been written about the ability of empaths to 'pick up' on other people's vibes. But I'm proposing something revolutionary – that we're *all* like a mobile phone that tunes in to other networks *automatically*.

Common Waves in Sync

This isn't a gift or a pathology that's reserved for extra-sensitive people (depending on how you look at it, of course). It applies to every single one of us. We not only 'capture' the energy of others,

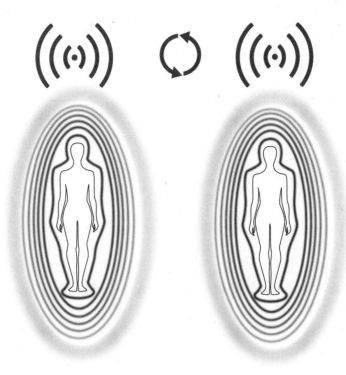

Human energy synchronization

we're also prone to forming a common 'wavelength' with them as part of our natural tendency to *synchronize* with each other.

This synchronization is a part of your inbuilt, default state of being: you were born with an inclination to tune in to another person's vibrations and auric waves! This hugely important understanding forms the foundation of my key principle for ensuring my patients achieve lasting health and avoid relapses.

Many of you will be aware that for thousands of years, healers have emphasized that humans don't live in splendid isolation, separate from the energy of our environment and other living organisms. I guess the most famous and popular ancient teaching on this subject, as I mentioned in the Introduction, is feng shui. It teaches us to harmonize the energy of our surrounding external space because doing so can benefit our wellbeing and improve the quality of our life.

Our social circle also forms a part of our environment, and we're all subconsciously adapting to it in one way or another. Many of us have spoken of finding a person's enthusiasm 'infectious', or felt that we've 'caught' someone's good mood. Equally, I imagine, we all know what it feels like to be in a 'negative' place or to be 'brought down' by someone.

We unconsciously synchronize with a friend's footsteps while out walking with them, or with the steady rhythm of the crowd when clapping along with fellow members of an audience. We are constantly seeking common ground so we can be in harmony with other people and our environment.

Fascinatingly, as we're about to discuss, modern science has already confirmed that the ability to tune in to each other emotionally, cognitively and physiologically is actually wired into us. Neurologists, linguists and biologists are publishing compelling evidence which demonstrates that naturally occurring physiological synchronicity – in which activity in the body over which we have no conscious control, such as brainwaves, heart rate, sweating and pupil dilation – is coordinated between two people.

This provides a completely new paradigm for viewing our social exchange with each other and our environment. It may help you to realize why, in the past, you might have been influenced by other people's vibrations and therefore failed to be your authentic self; and why it's so important to maintain your energy hygiene in the surrounding world of waves and vibrations.

I want to stress that although this discovery isn't something we should feel uneasy about, it does highlight the need to manage our energy in such a way that our energy ID stays intact. Otherwise, we'll be turned into sponges – absorbing all sorts of vibrational 'clutter' around us; or our inner state will always be dictated by the energy of other people or our environment. In this book, I'm going to show you how to own, rather than lose, your energy.

Science Fact Not Fiction

You might find the idea that you synchronize with other people's auras unbelievable – like something out of a sci-fi movie – but I'll shortly be introducing you to some thought-provoking scientific studies that encourage us to refresh our attitudes towards our connection with other people.

MRI scans reveal that our brainwaves cohere with those of other people; ECGs show that when we have an emotional connection with someone our heartbeats synchronize; and blood tests reveal that our hormonal balance can be influenced by the hormones of others. So, this is compelling evidence that we're not as autonomous as we once thought, and that we're united through our mutually created 'waves'.

However, this shouldn't automatically mean losing our energy ID and allowing others' waves to overpower our unique frequency. We can and should maintain our energy ID; however, as in any connection, it's vital that we have an awareness of the Self, in order to develop the trust that we are 'enough' just the way we are, and to cultivate healthy boundaries.

If we don't do this, we'll develop a codependency with others' energy, as happens in a destructive codependent romantic relationship. This will lead to unhealthy auric 'clinginess' and a susceptibility to toxic energy, and our sense of fulfilment and identity will depend on the approval or the emotional/mental state of other people.

Let's look a little closer now at the scientific evidence for synchronization and at the bonds that are formed between humans.

The Social Animal

Humans are social animals: we need to feel that we 'belong' to others and that we're connected. We live in groups, whether that's a family, a flat share, a wider social circle or as colleagues in an office. We care for our offspring for years and we cooperate with each other. Above all, we form lasting relationships with other individual humans – known by biologists as 'long-term pair bonds'. That's a rather formal description of what we usually call a romantic relationship; however, I think we also form a similar type of bond with people from our wider social circle.

Pair Bonds

According to biologists, humans create two main types of pair bond: one is social and the other is sexual. In the social pair bond there are strong behavioural and psychological links between two people, and their connection goes deeper than that of acquaintances. However, there's no sexual chemistry between them.

A sexual pair bond, meanwhile, involves strong behavioural and psychological links between two people; and of course there's also a powerful sexual attraction that usually develops into an exclusive sexual relationship. Interestingly, these pair bonds aren't restricted to humans: they are found in a variety of other species too.[1,2]

Our pair bonds with our fellow human beings affect our biology because they stimulate the production of various neurotransmitters, including oxytocin and dopamine. Oxytocin is sometimes called the 'love hormone' because it affects our emotions and social behaviour. For instance, we produce it during sex, and also when we hug someone because we're happy to see them. Dopamine helps to control the reward and pleasure centres in the brain, thereby affecting our mood.

Of course, some pair bonds are healthier than others. In a healthier bond, we feel good when we're with someone. We might even say that we're both 'on the same wavelength' or that we feel happy when we're with them. In biological terms – and I realize this is a very clinical way of describing what's going on between two people – each person is regulating the other's production of a whole range of different neurotransmitters. So when you're with someone who makes you feel good, your body is biologically synchronizing with theirs at a neurological and hormonal level.

Enjoying a healthy and deep connection with others not only regulates our nervous and hormonal systems through all the biological mechanisms of pair bonding, it also nourishes and uplifts our aura. When two auras with a similar frequency connect, it will always have an uplifting effect on us. It helps us to live longer, and it even regulates our heart and breathing rates, as I will explain later in this chapter.

Oh, Baby

The very first relationship we have as a baby is with our mother, while we're still in the womb. When many women give birth, their first instinct is to hold their newborn baby and look deeply into its eyes. Fathers of babies do this too, of course, when handed the new baby to hold.

This eye-to-eye contact is an instinctive reaction to the arrival of the new member of the family, but amazingly, it's also an opportunity for the brains of the parent and baby to synchronize, causing increased neural activity in both the adult and the child. Singing and talking to a baby while looking directly into its eyes, which is another natural parental instinct, also stimulates the child's neural activity. What's more, a baby will make more vocal sounds in return when an adult is making direct eye contact with it than when the adult isn't looking at it.[3]

This isn't the only form of synchronization that's taking place. The heart rhythms of the mother and baby are coordinated within less than one second when they start playing together, and this synchrony is even stronger when the mother speaks to her child.[4]

Attachment Theory

This is a theory that was developed in the 1950s by John Bowlby, an English psychiatrist, and Mary Ainsworth, an American psychologist, who conducted extensive studies into the relationship between a mother and her child. They found that if the mother isn't available for some reason, the primary caregiver fulfils her role instead.

Bowlby and Ainsworth believed that the quality of this mother–child link has a fundamental impact on the child's emotional development, setting the template for its future relationships, its ability to cope in the world and the development of its personality.[5]

When a baby is born, the adults who care for it regulate its life by feeding it, cuddling it and talking to it. At this stage, although the baby has the ability to experience and show deep emotions, it can't yet control the way it expresses these feelings, as you'll know all too well if you've ever been near a baby who is screaming for food or having a tantrum! If the baby has a reliable and committed relationship with one loving person, who is usually its mother, it will learn how to regulate its emotions.

The mother tunes in to her baby's material and emotional needs and then responds accordingly, thereby creating a healthy attachment. Conversely, an unhealthy attachment will arise if the mother is not fully engaging and communicating with her baby, is being unreliable, or is preoccupied with other things. Interestingly, in a healthy attachment, the mother and baby are almost turning into a synchronized system, and they both experience positive emotions. (We'll be exploring synchronization later in this chapter.)

A baby whose needs aren't being met by its mother, or main caregiver, becomes distressed, which increases its heart rate, breathing and blood pressure, and then sets off a chain reaction of stress hormones in its brain.[6] If this state continues, the baby shuts off from the world around it and retreats emotionally, as though it wants to become invisible.[7] If these stressful periods continue, disengaging from the world becomes a habitual part of the baby's coping strategy. What's more, these stressful episodes can even prevent the baby's brain from developing in certain ways.[8]

It isn't only babies who benefit from having a loving, secure and trusting relationship with their mothers. Toddlers need this as well, and it's only by the age of four that a child becomes more comfortable with the idea of being separated from its mother.[9,10] Even adolescents rely on a healthy attachment bond with their mother or other caregiver, even though by that time they may not always show it because they're learning to detach from their families and become more independent.

Don't imagine that the role of creating a healthy attachment bond with a baby rests entirely with the mother. The father or partner, as well as siblings and other members of the family, not to mention family friends, all play a vital role in helping the baby (and later, the child) to make emotional connections and to feel supported and loved.

Attachment Theory and the Aura

I find attachment theory fascinating because it chimes so well with what I know from the perspective of our aura, and from my healing work with my patients. When we're in our mother's womb our base chakra is dormant and we rely on our mother's base chakra instead. This means that the state of our mother's energy, healthy or otherwise, during her pregnancy has a huge impact on the development of our aura.

As soon as the umbilical cord that links us with our mother is cut after our birth, our base chakra is immediately activated. However, an invisible 'energy cord' that runs between our mother's navel chakra and ours will stay in place until we're between nine and 10 years old. I often tell my patients that they may be pregnant physically for nine months but they'll still be pregnant with their baby's spirit for the next nine or 10 years. (We'll be looking at energy cords in more detail later.)

This means that we as caregivers must take extra care of our aura because our baby/child will continue to tune in to our frequency and will rely on it for their own aura development. As attachment theory demonstrates, we must place our baby in a socially active environment so that he or she will develop in a healthy psychological atmosphere, and this also applies to the baby's energy development.

This kind of attunement, responsiveness and reaction to other human beings and their auras will continue throughout our lives. If you had a healthy energy development during your formative years you'll be primed to commit to a healthy energy exchange with other people.

However, if you had a negative mother–baby attachment, unless you're very aware of the effects this had on you and have taught yourself to be conscious of your behaviour, you might be prone to going into an energy-grabbing vampire state in which you use the energy of others; we'll be looking at energy vampires later. Alternatively, you might go to the opposite extreme of over-pleasing others and constantly sacrificing your energy, rather than engaging in the give and take of a healthier energetic flow.

Brain–Brain Connections

Did you know that your brain is directly affected by what you see other people doing? You might think that while you're relaxing and watching someone else being busy, you're being passive, but it turns out that this isn't what's happening at all.

Neuroscientists have studied what they call 'mirror neurons' in humans, chimpanzees and other primates. These neurons are cells that are activated whenever we perform a specific movement, such as reaching out to pick up a cup of tea. What makes mirror neurons so remarkable is that they are also activated when we see someone else making that same movement. So if you watch your friend reach out to pick up her cup of tea, thus activating her mirror neurons, the mirror neurons in *your* brain are also being activated. In other words, your brain has synchronized with your friend's.[11,12] You've no control over this – you're doing it unconsciously.

People working together in a close-knit team, all doing something at which they are expert, also experience a type of synchronization. I suppose you could say that they're all in the flow. The key regions and networks in the brain that are involved in performing such tasks show patterns of neural activity that are synchronized between all the members of the team, even if the actual movements they're making are quite different. This type of synchronization has been found in conversations, too, even when one person is speaking and the other is listening.[13]

Researchers have discovered that this type of synchronization applies in all sorts of situations, from two pilots sitting in a plane's cockpit[14] to people simply gazing into each other's eyes.[15]

Close Connections

We often refer to engaging in heart-to-heart conversations, or having heartfelt feelings for someone, and these aren't mere figures of speech. Our heart really is connecting with another person's. When we feel a deep emotional connection with someone, our heart will beat in time with theirs.[16] In other words, our two hearts synchronize. Think of all those songs and poems about two hearts beating as one.

The more we trust someone, the more likely it is that our heart rate will synchronize with theirs.[17] When we're involved in a romantic relationship, our heart and breathing rates can synchronize with our partner's, even when we aren't speaking or touching.[18,19] This isn't something we can control – it happens of its own accord.

Fascinatingly, we experience other physical effects over which we have no conscious control when we feel a deep connection with someone. For instance, if you're listening to a friend telling you a story and you're completely involved in what they're saying, the pupils in your eyes and those in your friend's eyes will contract and dilate in unison, in accordance with what's being said.[20]

Another amazing thing happens when you're talking to someone, even when you don't have a close rapport with that person. Every time you make a specific sound while talking, a tiny area in the prefrontal cortex in your brain is activated. There's an area like this for each of the different speech sounds that you make in your particular language. That same area will light up in the other person's brain, even though they aren't speaking at that point. This type of synchronization is the mechanism that allows us to hear speech sounds, and some scientists have even said that language is just a way for our brains to synchronize with each other.[21,22,23]

Have you ever noticed that when you're talking to a close friend you start to use the same sorts of words as they do, and that the rhythm of your speech becomes more like theirs? This is known as 'accommodation'. But it doesn't only happen between friends: it occurs every single time we talk to someone. As the conversation progresses, we begin to talk at the same speed and volume; we start to use the same words in the same way and our accents even start to sound more alike.[24,25]

As with other forms of synchronization, this isn't deliberate and we usually aren't even aware of it, but it has huge effects on us nonetheless. Accommodation makes us listen to each other, take each other seriously, and even agree with each other, and all of this happens without us knowing what's going on.[26] Of course, this is wonderful for creating a rapport with someone, but it also explains why we can be swayed by what people say even when we weren't interested in it at first.

It's Our Hormones

Hormones are chemicals in our blood that help to control many biological functions, including our brain activity, circulation, breathing, alertness and sexual arousal. It's also been known for a long time that hormones help to influence the empathy we have for one another.

But how does this work? It turns out that our empathy is affected by the synchronous increases and decreases in the levels of key hormones in our blood. Over long periods of time, our hormonal changes tend to become synchronized with those of the people we live with. For instance, it's long been known that women who live together all tend to menstruate at the same time each month because their cycles become synchronized.

These synchronous increases and decreases in the levels of some hormones are partly caused by the normal rise and fall of hormone levels during the day, but our hormones are synchronized with those of our romantic partner in other ways too. Researchers found that if a couple in a relationship go into a laboratory and one is put into a stressful environment, their stress-related hormones will spike. And so will their partner's, even though they aren't sharing that difficult environment.[27]

Animal Magic

There has already been a lot of research into the benefits on our blood pressure of petting and stroking animals,[28] but it's now being discovered that spending time with a cherished animal can also stimulate the production of beneficial hormones. Recent research shows that this happens between a human and their dog if they have a close relationship. If you're a dog owner, this may not come as a surprise to you!

One study found that when human handlers help their dogs to race through obstacle courses at competitive events, each human–dog pairing tends to experience exactly the same increases in blood levels of a specific hormone at exactly the same time.[29] Something similar happens between therapy dogs and their handlers who, of course, need to create a very close relationship if it's to be productive. If the handler gets upset, the dog (in its own canine way) experiences its owner's emotions through a synchronized increase in its own mood-related hormones.[30]

Another study explored the levels of oxytocin that are released in dog owners when they're reunited with their dogs after being away at work all day. If you have a dog, you'll know how delighted it is to see you when you walk through the door. Its body is flooded with pleasure-inducing hormones. But how does your body react? The study explored whether petting and stroking a dog stimulates our production of oxytocin, the 'love hormone'. Women reunited with their dogs had the highest increase in oxytocin production, although it's not yet known why.[31]

If you have a dog, do you kiss it? If you do, you might be interested to know that this raises your oxytocin levels, and it also raises your dog's. Well, that might seem obvious if you both enjoy showing affection for each other, but this isn't all that's happening. It seems that there are correlations between the oxytocin levels of both you and your dog during these sessions.[32] In other words, your oxytocin levels and those of your dog have synchronized.

More Senses Than You Know

Some people doubt my ability to detect the human energy field as it does require an extra sense beyond the five traditional ones – sight, sound, smell, touch and taste. However, let me surprise you by proving that you too have at least one more organ of perception than you previously thought.

Sit or stand comfortably, close your eyes and then touch the tip of your nose with your little finger. Now ask yourself a question – 'Which of the five senses enabled me to do that?' Yes, touch allowed your finger to make contact with your nose, but what was it that guided your finger to hit the right spot when your eyes were closed and you couldn't see what you were doing?

This is something called proprioception, which is your body's automatic ability to sense its position, motion and balance. It goes beyond each of the individual five senses. Examples like this one prove this, and encourage us to open our minds to the possibility that there's more to us that we realize.

The Aura and the Electromagnetic Field

Both our body and our aura are electromagnetic in nature. The cells in the human body are made up of electrons, protons, neutrons and other subatomic particles that, like everything else in the Universe, are always in a state of vibratory motion. When these particles vibrate, an electromagnetic radiation is emitted, which results in the formation of an electromagnetic field around our body.

In addition to the above we have tiny electrical currents running through our body due to the chemical reactions that occur as part of our normal bodily functions. For example, nerves relay signals by transmitting electrical impulses. Most biochemical reactions, from digestion to brain activities, go along with the rearrangement of charged subatomic particles.

Even the heart is electrically active – an activity that your doctor can trace with the help of an electrocardiogram. We all know from school that whenever there's an electric current, a magnetic field is produced. Interestingly, the heart's electrical field is about 60 times greater in amplitude than the electrical activity generated by the brain.[33]

The Eyes Have It

I'm convinced that science has yet to discover further evidence of our sensitivity to electromagnetic energy. For instance, we humans are able to sense light in more ways than one. Most of the time we rely on our visual sensitivity to light. The retina in the back of the eye contains two sorts of photosensitive cells that respond directly to electromagnetic stimulation. Rods respond to shape and motion, and cones respond to wavelength, which is what we call 'colour'.

When light hits the eye, the rods and cones transform that light into electromagnetic signals that travel down the optic nerve and into the brain, allowing us to sense colours, shapes and movement. We experience this as vision.

The human retina also contains a type of photoreceptor called a cryptochrome. When we're exposed to specific wavelengths of light, proteins called flavins gradually change their chemical structure and attach themselves to the cryptochromes, triggering a chemical reaction that in itself causes the slow build-up of a chemical called semiquinine. When enough semiquinine has been created, it produces an electrochemical response in the cryptochromes.

Here's where it gets really interesting. The brain receives this response and it activates various proteins that are crucial to the functioning of our circadian rhythms – physical, mental and behavioural changes in the body, including the speed at which our heart beats, the levels of adrenalin and other compounds in our blood, and the sensitivity of our nerves – that run in roughly 24-hour cycles. These cycles are controlled by our biological clocks and, as I've just explained, some of them are influenced by the activity of the cryptochromes in our eyes.

In other words, our eyes 'see' the time of day with the help of the subtle photoreceptors in our eyes, rather than with our vision. If you've ever felt wide awake after spending all evening on your computer, it's because the blue light emitted by its screen has activated the flavins in your eyes, which in turn have activated the cryptochromes, which have confused your biological clocks, which now think it's daytime rather than late evening!

It's not only humans who have cryptochromes in their eyes. Fascinatingly, in common birds such as the European robin, the cryptochrome proteins react with blue light and a molecule called flavin adenine dinucleotide, or FAD, which makes both molecules respond to the Earth's magnetic fields. Birds use this to navigate their way around. The big question is whether the cryptochromes in our eyes allow us to do the same thing.

Of course, we may not have the necessary electrochemical links in our brains to read what the sensors in our eyes are telling us. On the other hand, perhaps we have. If we do (and remember that proprioception proves that we have remarkable ways of combining our senses), it could be a sign of our own magnetic energy fields, and of the fact that we're biologically adapted to be sensitive to magnetic lines and their detection. Although much more scientific research is needed to prove these theories, there are indications that we humans – as well as birds – have more than one type of awareness.

Resonance and Vibration

I'm about to describe two of the fundamental laws of the Universe. Once you're familiar with them, you'll find it easy to understand – and, most importantly, to accept – that everything in the Universe is linked. In fact, when you consider the ways that these laws work in combination with each other, you'll realize that everything is connected at a *vibrational* level.

The Law of Vibration

This universal law has a profound connection to all that I'm telling you about in this book. The Law of Vibration states that when *everything* that exists in the Universe – including us – is broken down into its basic form, it consists of pure energy. And this energy is *vibrating* at various frequencies. Or, as *The Kybalion*, a guide to the teachings of a legendary sage has it: 'Nothing rests; everything moves; everything vibrates.'

It isn't just matter that vibrates energetically. Each thought, emotion and feeling we have and every word we speak, and each action intended and performed, also carries a charge of energy with its own matching vibrational frequency.

When I think about human vibrations, I use a formula:

**Thoughts + Feelings + Beliefs + Actions
+ Intention = Our Vibration**

Each part of this formula can alter our vibrations to a *higher frequency* – which is associated with good health, joy, and enlightenment – or regress it to a *lower frequency*, which is associated with illness, self-distraction and dark moods.

You need to understand your own vibration and its frequency if you're to take control of, and responsibility for, your life and wellness. Good health, happiness and abundance are 'high-frequency' states, so to resonate with them we must change the frequency at which we vibrate. Your own particular vibration acts as a magnet, so if you're troubled or worried, you'll attract toxic energy and will receive the very thing you're fearing.

If we focus on positive, high-frequency thoughts, feelings, actions, and intentions – such as love, gratitude and goodness – we'll increase these resonances in our body and strengthen it in very powerful ways. Conversely, if we focus on negative, 'low-frequency' emotions and states – such as hate, fear and division – we'll amplify those resonances in our body, and that will have a very harmful impact on us. As the Buddha told us: 'What you think, you become. What you feel, you attract. What you imagine, you create.'

It's also important to mention that each of us has our own 'vibrational radius'. People who have high-frequency vibrations and a wide vibrational radius are commonly described as charismatic. We feel inspired and uplifted in their presence. Later, I'll explain how you can establish daily high-frequency routines so you can raise your own vibrations.

The Law of Resonance

It may be a while since you studied physics, but what I'm about to tell you will give you a greater understanding of the energy concepts in this book. As you now know, there's no solidity in the Universe – everything in nature, including our thoughts, feelings and actions, is vibrating at a particular frequency.

The Law of Resonance states that when one object vibrates at the same frequency as a *second* object, that second object is forced into 'vibrational motion'. So when we talk about being in harmony with each other, we might think it's meant metaphorically, but in fact it's really happening – at a vibrational level.

The human energy field (the aura) and physical body behave in a similar way to the vibrating strings on a musical instrument: they will resonate to an internal or external stimulus – just like a tuning fork. The stimulus being introduced can be anything – a person, place or object – that carries a unique frequency, and which is part of a larger field of energy. Everything in the Universe has its own energy 'imprint' with a unique vibrational motion and a specific frequency.

Our energy reacts in order to adjust (resonate) to an external stimulus (other people, our environment, or external influences in general). We can experience this as feeling off-kilter, or it will resonate with our unique frequency, making us feel on top of things. This is one of the reasons why it's so important to look after and raise our frequency. The strong resonance of our energy with its authentic frequency is absolutely essential for our wellbeing. It's what I call living at peace with ourselves.

Finding Our Tribe

Let's return to the stringed instrument analogy. When an instrument's strings are strummed or plucked, they create vibrations that make sound waves. But it's not only stringed instruments that do this – everything that moves creates waves.

Now I'm going to tell you something fascinating about how these waves behave when they're in the same place at the same time. If two waves that share the same frequency travel in the same direction, and are identical to each other, they create one bigger wave. Science calls this 'constructive interference'. However, if those same two waves differ because one goes up at the point where the other goes down, they cancel each other out and there's no resulting wave. This is known as 'destructive interference'.

I think this is a perfect illustration of my belief that if we view ourselves as a unique 'wave' of energy (and the Law of Vibration allows us to do that), it's very important that we surround ourselves with people with whom we can connect or 'click'. In other words, we need to find our tribe. When we do that, the resulting constructive interference means we amplify each other. However, the reverse happens when we're with people who aren't on our wavelength for some reason. Rather than positive amplification, we create destructive interference, which leads to a significantly weaker energy field.

BECOME A TUNING FORK

This is a very useful meditation that will help you to reflect on the frequency and vibrations you radiate, which are dependent on your emotional and mental state. It's not a very glamorous idea, but you're going to imagine yourself as a big tuning fork. Be sure to practise this at a time (and in a place) when you won't be disturbed.

Sit comfortably in a chair or in your favourite meditation pose. Take three deep breaths and feel yourself relaxing. Close your eyes.

Picture yourself as a human tuning fork, and think carefully about what you're attracting into your life. Bear in mind that whatever you attract will amplify within you, and these are the frequencies you'll be emitting. Make no judgement about what you've been attracting – just observe it and make a mental note.

Now that you've done this, you can conduct a seven-day experiment in which you meditate for a short time every day and focus on cultivating the inner states of love, gratitude and kindness. The energy of these emotions is high frequency, and it will have the same uplifting effects on your vibrations.

At the end of the week, observe what has changed in your life. Even better, write down these changes, so you can refer back to them whenever you need to remind yourself of the power of your thoughts.

. . . .

If you enjoyed this meditation, you can continue with it. Perhaps it will be the start of a life-enhancing new habit or a daily high-frequency routine.

Are You Receiving Me?

Every one of us emits and receives energy all the time. Our bodies do it automatically, in many different physiological ways, as you've already learned. But this isn't all that's happening. We emit and receive energy at an emotional and mental level too. It's an integral part of being alive.

An easy way to understand this is to think about a car radio, which tunes in to a radio station whenever it moves into its transmission range. Would you be surprised to learn that you're doing exactly the same thing, all the time? You're always picking up the frequencies that surround you, whatever you're doing – whether it's watching TV at home, being at work, taking your child to school, chatting to a friend, or any of the other many activities you're involved in. The frequencies that you encounter are being transmitted to you, and you too are transmitting your own frequencies.

And, in the same way that you enjoy listening to some radio stations and dislike others, you'll have the same kinds of reactions to the frequencies you're picking up throughout the course of each day. Some of these frequencies will be instant new favourites, and you'll want to add them to your metaphorical playlist, while others may take a bit of getting used to.

For instance – continuing with the car radio analogy – you might be a big fan of classical music but your radio tunes in to a hard rock station. It's not what you'd choose to listen to but you decide to give it a try anyway. You may be surprised to find that you enjoy it, or it may eventually get on your nerves because it sounds so discordant, making you lose your inner sense of harmony. And some of the stations you pick up might even be an immediate no-no, so you'll want to switch over as soon as you can.

One of the key ideas I'd like to convey to you is that we should only allow ourselves to tune in to what we're comfortable with. However, it's good to stretch ourselves a little and see if we like something we've never come across before, but if we decide it's not for us, we need to move on. If that's not possible, we need to find a way of disengaging from whatever it is we don't like.

CHAPTER 4

Energy Pollution in Your Environment

We can all feel the energy that surrounds us, even when we aren't consciously aware of it. We feel good when we're with someone who has uplifting energy because they give our energy a boost. We might feel happier and lighter when we're with them, or more optimistic; or perhaps the problem we've been worrying about no longer feels like such a burden and we start to see ways to resolve it.

It works the other way around too, of course. When we approach a hostile-looking gang of people in the street, we're affected by their energy as we hurry past. We'll probably have some physical reactions: for instance, our stomach might contract into a tight knot of anxiety, the hairs on the back of our neck might start to prickle, or we might sense that we're being watched by these individuals who seem so threatening.

If you've ever visited someone who was ill, maybe in a hospital or a care home, you may recall that the experience affected you in ways that were hard to put into words. Maybe you felt anxious about that person and were upset to see them suffering. That's a perfectly natural reaction, but perhaps you also struggled to shake off those feelings afterwards. It was as though they became stuck to you – like white dog hair on a black jacket, or like a lingering, bad aftertaste – and it took you a while to get rid of them. Or maybe you've never quite managed to get over that experience, and it still haunts you sometimes.

The same thing can happen even when you're not directly involved in what you're witnessing. For instance, have you ever started to cry while watching a tragic story unfolding on the TV news? Have you ever woken in the middle of the night, your stomach churning as you remember all too vividly the disturbing scene in the book you were reading just before you turned out the light? Or have you ever found yourself spending hours going over and over in your mind a row you had with your partner, keeping alive all the anger and hurt you felt at the time while feeling powerless to do anything about it?

Soon I'll be teaching you all sorts of techniques to help you deal with situations like these, so you can reclaim your energy now and learn how to protect it in the future. I'm also going to tell you about the areas of your life that are stealing your energy, even if you're unaware that's happening.

Energy Abuse

We're all strongly affected by the energy of the people around us. Unfortunately, this can become as much of a vicious circle as the disease-cure-reinfection cycle I described earlier. 'Mutual energy abuse' happens to many of us all the time. For instance, how often have you come home from a difficult day and taken out your frustration, anxiety or anger (or all three) on the people around you? Maybe you couldn't stop yourself snapping at your child or your partner when they asked you a simple question.

Alternatively, perhaps you're often on the receiving end of someone else's bad mood, which can set the scene for a blazing row or for one of you to burst into tears and storm out of the room. Then, during mealtimes, you might suffer from indigestion because you're still feeling so irritated or annoyed by what happened that your digestive system cannot process your food. You simply can't 'stomach' the bad day or negative event. And so it goes on...

The words we use when talking about ourselves to others, or in our head, can be abusive, too, even if we don't realize it. I think of them as auric graffiti because they scribble themselves all over our aura, pollute it and sidetrack our energy with negative labels, and if we don't know they're present we can't clear them away. Once you start paying attention to all this auric graffiti you'll hear it everywhere. It's endemic.

TV programmes can be full of negativity too. Docusoaps in particular often focus on people's problems. I'm sure you know the sort of thing I mean – shows about how unhappy an individual is, or about their bizarre health problem; or the terrible things that have happened to people and how they're apparently trapped in a dead-end situation with no solution in sight. TV dramas, not to mention films, often dwell on frightening situations, with menacing or psychopathic characters who prey on everyone around them. Yet strangely, we think this is suitable viewing when we curl up on the sofa and relax after a hard day!

Often we don't even notice the negative messages that these films and TV programmes are sending us, because we've become anaesthetized to them. Or we think we have... Our auras tell a different story, though. Such repetitive exposure to negativity creates a template for our aura but it's not one that's healthy or positive.

In the same way, when we're constantly replaying in our mind's eye negative events from our past, and feeding off old problems, it isn't good for our health. Pay particular attention if you tend to 'recycle' the energy of the past in this way when you're ill, as this is not conducive to recovery. I see this as a bleak position to be in because it's always focusing on the negative.

Carrying Negative Baggage

I'm always amazed at the way some of us tend to immerse ourselves in negativity without even being aware of it. When you're walking down the street and you step in some dog poo, you won't leave it on your shoes for a minute longer than necessary, and you certainly won't announce to everyone what happened or pull more people towards the mess. You'll probably rush to scrape it off on some grass or on the side of the pavement, and then you'll thoroughly wash your shoes and feet as soon as you can. You'll remove every speck of the mess until you feel clean again and you can no longer smell it.

Yet it's often a completely different story when we step in metaphorical dog poo in the shape of something negative or upsetting happening to us. Instead of doing what we can to get rid of it as fast as possible, we tend to stay trapped in that stench of negativity. We might even brood on it or drag more people inside it, replaying it over and over in our mind, rather than switch off from it or do something to improve the situation.

This means that whenever we encounter some negative energy we must train ourselves not to dwell on it. We need to get rid of it in a positive way so we can immediately feel better and don't use it as an excuse to vent our emotions on the people around us.

Please understand that what I'm talking about here are the everyday problems that can spring up between people – all those niggles and arguments and crossed wires. Sometimes we all have to deal with really difficult or unhappy situations, such as relationship break-ups and bereavements, and it's bound to take us longer to cope and come to terms with them. But even then, the focus shouldn't be on dwelling but on a proactive forward process of healing.

In Parts 5 and 6 I'll be showing you how you can become alert to these negative energies and how you can protect your aura from them; you'll also learn ways to cleanse your aura of negative energies if you think they've attached themselves to you. When you understand the harm that this type of energy can do, you'll realize that they aren't something you want stuck to your aura. Actually, it's often not an event or an emotion that's affecting us but our dwelling on something that makes us miserable or angry.

You'll also come to realize that it's essential for you to take responsibility for your own energy and how you use it. You need to ensure as much as possible that you don't pass to other people your own anger or bad mood or fear or negative energy. If you don't stop yourself from doing this, you'll be part of the problem rather than part of the solution. And besides, it will cause them harm, just like passive smoking. You must be more loving and considerate towards the people around you, and protect them from your toxic fumes!

Energy Thieves

Here's a very important point for you to think about, because it's one of the common reasons why people sabotage their wellness and healing treatments: before you contemplate ways to increase your energy and vitality, you must work out *how* you're *losing* your energy in the first place. Otherwise, it's like putting money into a pocket with a hole in it.

We tend to focus on topping up our energy reserves and neglect our multiple energy leaks. But if we stop and think about it, it's pretty silly to complain about our depleted 'energy banks' without ever wondering what and who is stealing energy from us. So it's important for you to identify the energy 'thieves' in your life, whatever they/it happen to be. And don't be surprised if that thief is actually *you!*

If you're a parent you might now be muttering to yourself that holding down a demanding job, bringing up your children and ferrying them round to all their after-school activities, juggling your finances and trying to shoehorn a social life into the remaining hours of the week is more than enough explanation for your constant tiredness.

But there could be other reasons for your sluggish energy or your longing to flake out on the sofa while the rest of the world leaves you in peace, and many of them happen without you even realizing it. Are you giving a lot of your energy away to someone with whom you're annoyed – by mentally rehashing all the things about them that make you so angry? Maybe you had a disagreement with someone on social media and have since been wishing you'd replied differently, even finding yourself gripped by anxiety when you think about it.

Or perhaps you're giving your energy to someone out of pity? We often give energy to others when we feel sorry for them, but then we don't give ourselves permission to moderate our generous energy offerings, even though they're draining us. Whenever you react to a situation like this, and have it running in your mind on a never-ending mental loop, you're keeping its energy alive and damaging your own in the process. Handing out your energy in this way will have a depleting effect on your aura.

And most importantly, don't forget that if you allow in an external energy that doesn't resonate with your unique energy ID, it will have a negative effect on you. Every time you commit to something that goes against you inner truth, it will rob you of energy.

We often choose to see people socially or keep them as friends even though we've grown out of resonance with them long ago. This can be a very expensive habit for our aura. You really need to think about your true, intuitive, reactions to the people you choose to spend time with, such as your friends and family. Ask yourself how they affect you. How they make you feel. I'm sure you'll find it very illuminating when you start to analyse your reaction to each friend and family member using the following exercise; this process shouldn't be rushed.

REFLECTING ON YOUR FAMILY AND FRIENDS

Set aside some time to sit quietly and peacefully by yourself to do this exercise. (Don't do it when there's someone else in the room with you because you might then be picking up on their energy, which will be confusing).

1. Begin with your friends. Imagine as vividly as possible each friend in turn standing next to you. It's important not to engage your mental judgement here, such as labelling the person 'good' or 'bad', or thinking things like, *she/he did so much for me* or *he/she went through so much in life*. Your reflection should be connected to the present and only involve your feelings at that given moment.

2. Stay present and listen to your *feelings*, not your mind. Where in your body do you register your reaction to each person, and how do you feel about them? For instance, imagining that one particular friend is next to you might give you a tingly and excited feeling in your chest, and you might even decide to call them when you've finished the exercise because you always love chatting to them.

When thinking about another friend, however, you might realize that your stomach has just done a little somersault and your energy has plummeted because you've remembered you're seeing them soon. What does this tell you about them, and about your reaction to them?

3. When you've worked your way through your friends, do the same thing with the members of your family.

Try to do this exercise as calmly as possible, and without judgement. You're not doing it to find fault with people or to remind yourself of previous clashes with them; instead, the aim is to discover how they affect your energy at the time of the exercise. You might also have some insights into how you can change things in the future.

Please note that I said how they affect your energy *at the time of the exercise*. Energy changes all the time, so it's helpful to do this exercise regularly; in this way you can monitor the feelings you get and adjust your boundaries accordingly. For instance, your reaction to some people might vary according to what's been happening between you or how you're feeling at the time, but you may always respond to other people in exactly the same way, whatever that happens to be.

Remember too, that the purpose of this exercise is not to label someone as 'good' or 'bad'. It's just a tool you can use to reflect on the true state of your energy connection, so you can adjust it if necessary. Just look at it as a 'wave check'.

. . . .

Be Clear Why You Want More Energy

Another reason why so many people live in a state of chronic energy deficiency, despite various attempts at finding a cure, is because deep down they don't know *why* they want to be well or to have more energy. When people give an honest answer to this question, they're often surprised to discover how much they're being driven by fear. For instance, they might say, 'I'm scared of suffering' or, if they're currently healthy, 'I don't want to become ill.'

Some people come to see me because a loved one has died after a chronic illness and they're frightened that the same thing will happen to them. Others have reached the halfway point in their life and are worried about ageing – terrified that it's going to be downhill from now on. Some of my patients read the endless health scare stories in the media, being told one week that a food is good for them and the next week that it's likely to shorten their lives. They don't know what to do for the best, and they gradually begin to believe that the world is an unsafe place – full of dangers and perils that they need to avoid.

Your motivation for wellness should be a positive one. Choose wellness rather than an escape from suffering! As we discussed earlier, fear is such a low-frequency emotion that it often attracts the very same things that we fear. Wellbeing should be your proactive choice.

Change, But Not Just Yet

Have you ever heard the joke about the person who prayed, 'Please God, make me good, but not just yet?' It's funny, but also acts as a reminder that some people ask for change even though, deep down, they aren't ready to accept it in the present moment.

This can happen in all sorts of ways. A person might desperately be praying for a cleaner, lighter body, but at the same time doesn't want to give up drunken late nights or a junk-food diet. Or it might be someone trying to attract a new, loving relationship while feeling reluctant to let go of a previous partner from whom they've grown apart. Someone else might ask for more energy while still wanting to carry on spending all day lazily watching TV in bed.

There are countless other examples when we're split between desperately wanting a change yet are reluctant to create space for it. You can't attract change with an intent to secure it and put it on hold for when it's more convenient. So if you're wishing for transformation, make sure you really want it *now* and are ready to receive it.

Energy Wastefulness

Another factor in the wellness deficit is a subconscious attachment to energy blockages or tiredness. This can become so integral to someone's identity that they cannot separate themselves from it. And in some cases a lack of vitality is used as a scapegoat for all of life's failures. It almost acts as a buffer between the person and life itself. Or it becomes a means of getting extra love and attention from others.

Other people actually embrace tiredness as a means of escaping their problems. In fact, this is a subliminal desire to disappear. They make themselves comfortably numb so they almost can't feel anything at an emotional or a mental level. And if we spend too much time with someone when they are in this state, we too become only partially charged with energy. We become dull or listless, especially if we're trying to motivate them to perk up while they are subliminally invested in benefiting from their lethargy.

Some people skip from one spiritual practice to another and are always searching for the light, but they never give themselves sufficient time to engage with one before they discard it and start looking for something else. Even though they are always looking for the light, they resemble a mole because they stay attached to the darkness. This drains their energy, and it becomes a vicious circle – subconsciously they keep sabotaging themselves into the convenient proof that darkness is more comfortable, but each pull-back makes them more tired than before.

And lastly, a very common mistake is the way we inadvertently use negative verbal statements when we're trying to attract better health and wellness. The subconscious mind doesn't understand the subtleties of negative statements so, for instance, instead of interpreting 'I don't want to become ill' as 'I want to remain healthy', it picks up on the words 'become ill' and delivers that outcome instead.

Equally, with 'I don't want to suffer any longer', it simply latches onto the word 'suffer' and provides more opportunities for suffering in the future. So, statements such as 'I choose health' or 'I'm committed to feeling better every day' have a lot more power to snap you out of your lethargy.

Once you've finished reading this chapter, spend some time reflecting on whether anything I've described applies to you. Be honest with yourself! Always remember the following points when you're trying to embark on change:

❖ Consider how you benefit from, and invest in, your current state.

❖ Be as honest with yourself as possible about *why* you're striving towards wellness.

❖ Choose positive active words when affirming what you intend to happen.

❖ Don't let yourself be driven by fear.

The Wellness Saboteurs

In the Prologue I touched on the concept of energy pathogens, which have a *toxic effect* on our aura and life. And in Part 2 you learned about the waves and vibrations that surround us and how our personal vibrations naturally tune in to them.

The toxic energy pathogens we'll be exploring in the next part of the book are really vibrations caused by the interference between incompatible energy fields. These vibrations manifest first of all in our personal space, but they can then travel inwards through the layers of our aura, straight towards our core.

I use the word 'toxic' because, just like a poison, the energy of these vibrations is dangerous to our life force and damaging to our wellbeing. They penetrate our aura and disrupt our energy ID, and rob us of the chance to live authentically. Besides, all pathogens, whether they are biological or energetic, are parasitic and take energy from the host they are occupying. So, this unseen world of energetic germs must be uncovered if we're to master the energy of our environment – something that's essential to protect our wellbeing.

As my gift allows me to sense all these energy pathogens, I feel I can share with you what I detect under the 'microscope' of my hands. I'm not pretending to give you a scientific analysis here; I just know that when I apply this knowledge in my practice it leads to profound changes. My patients, once equipped with these insights, always report that their new awareness dramatically improves their quality of life.

I don't want anyone to become mired in ignorance, in the way that our ancestors did, and suffer as a result of something that can be easily prevented. I hope that science will eventually verify my hypotheses about energy pathogens and the energy exchange between humans, but until then all the information I'm about to give you bears the evidence of my years as a successful energy healer.

While working with my patients I've been struck by the similarity between the way our body is penetrated by biological pathogens and the mechanism by which our aura is penetrated by energy 'germs'. In fact, the methods of infiltration used by the latter are almost identical to those used by biological bacteria, viruses and fungi.

Interestingly, we can be affected by toxic vibrations in our external environment and also by those we generate ourselves, in one of the layers of our aura. This is a very important point because the majority of people tend to look outside themselves to find the cause of negative energy. Owning our energy always entails taking responsibility for it. So, before pointing the finger at someone and blaming them for our problems, we should first examine ourselves and see where we may be harbouring and cultivating toxic parasitic entities within us.

So, let's now dive deep into the fascinating world of energy pathogens, what I call auric 'bacteria', auric 'viruses' and auric 'fungi'.

Part III

THE
THREE
ENERGY
PATHOGENS

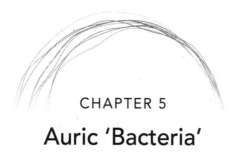

CHAPTER 5

Auric 'Bacteria'

In this chapter, I'm going to introduce you to auric 'bacteria', but before I tell you how they manifest and infiltrate our aura, I want to describe what bacteria are in biological terms. Bacteria are simple microorganisms – living cells that thrive in all sorts of environments both inside and outside humans and other living beings. Bacteria can happily survive without a host and reproduce on their own, but they do require specific environmental conditions, which can be living or decaying organisms.

The important point to remember about bacteria is that they don't infiltrate and inject their DNA into our cells. Instead, bacteria are cells that *co-exist* with ours: they simply use us as their environment.

So, what are auric 'bacteria'? These are energy vibrations that intrude into our aura but don't alter our unique frequency. In other words, they don't change *our* energy ID by projecting *their* energy ID but simply consume our energy resources. As a result of these interactions, we become drained and our wellbeing suffers. Most frequently, auric 'bacteria' enter our aura through its emotional layer.

Energy Cords

As you now know, when we connect with someone our auras move together and produce a common 'wave' of energy. In largely healthy connections these waves are fluid, light and non-binding: they allow the energy between two people to flow equally, without dominance or one-sided pressure.

Earlier I explained that some of these common energy waves are temporary and act as an important mechanism for our survival, as in the case of a healthy attachment between mother and child. Sadly, other waves are simply parasitic and damaging, because a person, just like a bacterium, starts to use you as their environment. Then, these common energy waves become rigid and cord-like, attaching that person to your energy field (aura) in order to pull your energy towards them.

Energy Cords in the Chakras

Often, these pathogen-like 'energy cords' latch onto you through your energy centres – your chakras. The following are the most common examples of how the energy cords manifest in the chakras.

Base Chakra

This is the chakra of survival, so an energy cord here is about someone needing you in order to survive. Of course, this is perfectly natural between a parent and child, but it isn't helpful when it occurs between two people in negative circumstances. For instance, it can happen when one work colleague uses another's energy and ideas to promote themselves.

Navel Chakra

An energy cord in this, the chakra of sexual and emotional intimacy, can be formed when someone regards you as a sexual object rather than a person in your own right. A cord can also form here when someone is completely dependent on your emotional support.

Solar Plexus Chakra

When there's an energy cord in this chakra, which generates energy in the body, it's almost as if one person has plugged into the other's energy stores, so they can draw on their persona and adopt their image.

Heart Chakra

People who share a deep love for each other will have a very powerful energy cord that links their two heart chakras. This can be a wonderfully positive experience, but, as with everything else in life, we must take responsibility for the effects it has on both parties. It can be life-enhancing and profoundly spiritual if both people feel the same way, but sometimes a cord can form here in the case of unrequited love, so that one person is imposing on the energy of the other.

Throat Chakra

Guilt can create a strong energy cord between people through this chakra. We can experience it almost viscerally and often describe guilt as 'suffocating'. An energy cord running to this chakra also means that the other person is too desperate to communicate with you; imposed words can also form cords in this chakra.

Third Eye Chakra

Energy cords form in this chakra, which governs clairvoyance and intuition, when one person cannot stop thinking about the other. Cords can also form between friends or partners if one party is always wondering what the other is thinking about.

Crown Chakra

The crown chakra rules true knowledge. When there's an energy cord hooking into this chakra, it can be because someone wants to impose their ideas on you or to manipulate you into doing as they say. The teachers in some occult schools have been known to deliberately create cords to their pupils' crown chakras, so they will be obedient and dutiful. Politicians can also create crown chakra energy cords with the public, in order to control their opinions.

Other Types of Energy Cord

I just want to add a couple more points. When a couple splits up, they may not see each other any more but the loving common energy wave between them often turns into a rigid cord that will continue to exist unless it's deliberately severed. This is also true for friendships that break down, or any other close relationship that comes to an end.

If you don't cut the cords between you and the other person, you can still have an energetic attachment to them, and this can lead to all sorts of imbalances on the mental and emotional levels and an inability to start a new relationship or friendships. You might feel as if that person still inhabits your space, and you're simply unable to open up to a new partner.

And lastly, I want to warn anyone in a caring profession, such as medics, therapists and carers, that if you're not careful with your professional boundaries – a subject we'll be discussing shortly – you will be forming energy cords with your patients. This is especially true if you tend to sacrifice yourself for your patients, rather than helping them. There is a difference... Or if you tend to work in a demanding environment in which patients attribute their ability to survive to you alone. This is also true for people who work in orphanages.

All these jobs are hugely admirable, and often the people who do them are true heroes, but I do hope they can benefit their own wellness by taking better care of their aura.

Promises, Promises

We have to be vigilant when making promises to others, especially if we do it out of guilt or because we feel we've been bullied into it. If this happens to you, the promise you made will create a very strong energetic connection between you and the other person, and your life force will be pulled towards them.

So take care when making a promise, especially if it puts you in the position of being someone's saviour or guardian. To give you an example, making the very profound promise to a friend or lover that 'I will always look after you' casts you in the role of their saviour. Are you sure that you want this? Of course, it's fine if you do, but often we make this kind of statement without any awareness of the repercussions for our energy field.

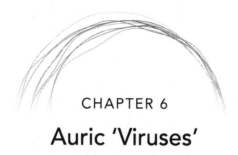

CHAPTER 6

Auric 'Viruses'

Unlike bacteria, biological viruses can only survive if they infiltrate a living cell. They bind to a cell in our body and then penetrate it, taking over the cell's inner mechanisms. The DNA of the virus becomes dominant, forcing our cell's own DNA to produce copies of the invading virus. I think we can almost call this cell hijacking!

Auric 'viruses' are the energy forms that break through our aura and take up residence inside us. Unlike auric bacteria, they *do* have the power to bend our unique energy ID to match *their* energy ID. We become compromised on an existential level, or on the level of self-identity.

Our unique frequency becomes enslaved by someone else's; and of course, this means that we completely lose the ability to live authentically. Often the auric 'virus' attacks us through a few layers of our aura simultaneously and particularly involves strong, order-like suggestions that infiltrate the mental layer. Our auric layers become 'decoded' so they match the nature of the intruder rather than our true self. Often this is done through verbal exchanges.

Sadly, we tend to forget that each thought we have and word we speak carries a charge of energy with its own matching frequency. So one example of an auric 'virus' is addressing each other in a negative way – this could be a put-down that someone repeats to us, over and over, until we believe what they're saying and start to feel inadequate.

Such verbal 'labels' eventually affect us so much that they deprogramme us. Our aura has been hacked and we start running someone else's programme instead of our own. This means we end up saying and doing things in the hope that we'll please this person, rather than because these actions reflect our authentic self. Or we just slowly, without even realizing it, mould ourselves into manifesting the self-image being imposed on us. We've caught an auric virus!

Living With Your 'Inner Troll'

But how about the negative messages we give ourselves? These are sent by something that I jokingly call our 'inner troll'. When we talk about trolls we're usually referring to the people who enjoy stirring up trouble on the Internet: posting provocative or aggressive comments on websites or social media platforms to get a reaction so they can enjoy watching the argument that erupts as a result. They thrive on this sort of attention and the mayhem they can create.

What we tend to overlook, though, is how often we act like trolls within ourselves. We often allow our inner chatter to 'self-hack' our aura by criticizing, belittling and second-guessing ourselves. This is a very common reason for the wellness self-sabotage I described earlier in the book, and why people fail to sustain any improvements made from the various therapies they explore.

It's very important that you don't allow your 'inner troll' to take control – if you do, it will start to undermine your confidence and make you doubt yourself. It might tell you that you can't do various things; that they're impossible and you might as well give up now. There are particular situations, especially those that put your self-confidence to the test and make you vulnerable, which can trigger that troll and amplify its voice, so you must learn how to manage them. Don't worry: I'll be giving you lots of advice on how to do this.

Dangerous Metaphors

You need to find ways to disable this negative self-programming, and one of them is to look at how you talk to yourself and describe your life to others. This is really important because the way you speak dictates the way you live. The energy of words is denser than the energy of thought, and it's therefore a big influence in our lives.

We must all avoid using aura-damaging words and metaphors. Very often, we aren't even aware of what we're saying because these words and phrases are so familiar to us. Yet we haven't understood their underlying meaning. They may be a part of our everyday language, but that doesn't prevent them from damaging our aura. When we use them, we're creating in the mental layer of our aura rigid templates that are reshaping and limiting our entire aura.

Here are some examples, although there are many, many more. Maybe you use some of them yourself, or hear other people using them.

❖ 'That's to die for.'

❖ 'No way! I'd rather stick pins in my eyes.'

❖ 'I can't stomach it a moment longer.'

❖ 'It was like a knife in my heart.'

❖ 'He makes me sick.'

❖ 'I'm feeling gutted.'

❖ 'I'm dead tired.'

❖ 'It chopped me off at the knees when that happened.'

❖ 'I'm going for a killer look.'

❖ 'It breaks my heart.'

❖ 'This job will finish me off.'

We think we're 'only' using metaphors here, but in fact we're giving our energy a command. As I've mentioned before, the unconscious doesn't know the difference between metaphor and reality. So when we say things like 'I'm sick to death of my job', we're creating the energetic template for disease.

It might take a while before you stop using phrases like these, especially if they are so ingrained that you've never realized what you're really saying. The good news is that you *can* stop using them. Once you begin to be conscious of the power of your words you'll find that you become increasingly aware of what you're saying, and you'll automatically start to choose more positive words and phrases. This will have a beneficial impact on your aura, and therefore on your mental and emotional outlook, and will make your personal vibration a lot stronger.

Verbal Handcuffs

Words and phrases can act like handcuffs, too. When we say things like 'I'll never be able to learn how to do that' or 'It's impossible', it causes our energy to stagnate. These might appear to be harmless phrases, and you might even think that you're simply stating a fact when you say something like, 'I could no more do that than fly to the Moon.' However, just as negative self-talk can damage your aura, so can phrases like these.

This is because when you dissect the statement 'I can't do it', it's all about *not* believing in yourself. You think that you aren't capable of doing something, or maybe you believe that you simply don't *deserve* to be able to do it. Of course, it could be that you really *can't* do something, but do check that this isn't just your default statement.

Another possibility is that you believe it doesn't matter what you want because other people's needs are more important than your own, and you have to go to the back of the queue. In other words, these phrases are acting like viruses, causing aura-squashing diseases that I call 'Limitation', 'Restriction' and 'Confinement'.

We all have our own ways of tripping ourselves up like this, so it's a question of discovering what your verbal weaknesses are, and then becoming more aware of them and more vigilant about avoiding them. For instance, try using positive phrases, such as 'I intend to...', 'I'm committed to...', 'I've decided...' and 'I'm determined to try...'. Don't just say them, though – *really believe* in what you're saying!

I often tell my patients: 'You can. And if you start, you will.' Learn to use words as wings rather than handcuffs.

Putting Yourself Down

Emphasizing something negative about yourself is another example of your 'inner troll' in action. For instance, many people are anxious about how they look and they unconsciously reinforce that through their choice of words. You need to check your language all the time and rephrase it whenever you realize you've said something negative. For instance, instead of telling yourself 'I'm so fat that I'll never fit into beautiful clothes', try 'I need a different size' or 'At the moment, another colour is more flattering.'

Another thing that lots of us do is undermine our intelligence. Have you ever picked up a book, thought the text looked really complicated, and said, 'Wow, I'm not clever enough to understand this'? It might seem that you're making a joke, and anyone listening might laugh with you. However, your unconscious doesn't have a sense of humour, so the message it's absorbing is that you're stupid and are prepared to remain that way.

Lastly, I want to mention a very common tendency to joke about our age. So many people are way too young to be concerned and embarrassed about their age, yet they joke about 'losing the face', about their 'creaking bones' or 'having dementia'. I'd encourage you to see statements like these not as funny phrases but as damaging and energy altering self-programming.

'I Am'

The word 'I' is very powerful, because it's so personal. When you say 'I' you're talking directly about yourself. This means that you need to be very careful about the statement you make *after* saying 'I am'. Try to avoid identifying with anything negative and limiting.

Sometimes a patient will come to me saying, 'Please help me, because I'm depressed.' Although this might seem a perfectly natural thing to say, it means they are identifying themselves with the state of being depressed. When you say 'I'm depressed', you *become* your condition. So, don't identify with your condition and don't become your diagnosis! Your illness is not *you*.

Instead of saying 'I'm depressed,' it's better to say 'I'm in a depressive state.' If you're unhappy, it's healthier to say 'I'm feeling sad' instead of 'I'm sad.' I'm sure you'll be able to come up with your own variations on this concept, according to your personal state. In another words, use these statements as descriptions of your *current* state rather than definitions of yourself.

Try also to avoid statements like 'I'm useless', 'I'm stupid', 'I'm fat', etc. Combinations of 'I am' with very low-frequency words certainly won't amplify your auric vibrations and they will seriously compromise your vitality.

Your Shadow

'A man who is possessed by his shadow is always standing in his own light and falling into his own traps ... living below his own level.' These are the words of Carl Jung, the Swiss psychoanalyst and founder of analytical psychology. He famously talked about the shadow, which he described as our subconscious 'dark side'. It is really a block to our best self and, in my mind, the place where our 'inner troll' resides.

You can think of the shadow as the ugly version of yourself. It's the side of you that you don't want to identify with, and which for various reasons you push down (often without realizing it) into your unconscious. There can be many facets to our inner shadow, depending on how many behaviours or qualities we choose to repress.

Rather than trying to control an aspect of ourselves that we can't handle, many of us prefer to push it away and pretend it doesn't exist. This means that we think we don't *have* to deal with it. This hidden part of us can still have a voice and be a very harsh critic, though, and it can eventually lead us towards self-sabotage and the destruction of our energy field. What's more, the smaller we consider ourselves to be and the more we doubt our inner light, the bigger our shadow becomes. This is why, in the previous chapters, I urged you to eradicate belittling inner self-talk and limiting self-beliefs.

Remember, we all have a shadow, so it's not the case that some people are perfect and others aren't. It's part of our make-up as human beings. Instead of denying it, we need to acknowledge it. After all, if we were pure light we'd be angels, not humans! So we need to accept the existence of our shadow and its 'trolling' force, but at the same time remember to stay in the state of a master and continue to enhance our inner light and keep on amplifying our unique frequency.

Of course, I approach shadow work as a healer, and I believe that we have to commit our lives to attracting more light, so it becomes our dominant force. Please remember that we're not seeking perfection here, but *authenticity*. Your authentic self will always radiate a stronger energy frequency than your perfect self. Besides, when I see people who are trying to appear perfect, they are the ones who have a huge but repressed shadow. Once again, the best way to reduce your shadow force is to work on uplifting your unique frequency, rather than simply hiding from your shadow. So be choosy about which internal voice you listen to. It's a question of what's your driving force and what you choose to be your driver.

There's a very good story from Jewish folklore that illustrates this perfectly. A snake's tail was having an argument with its head. The tail complained to the head, saying, 'You always lead, you always go first, and I'm fed up with it.' The head replied, 'OK, you go first, then.' And of course the blind tail led the snake to some nearby bushes covered in thorns that ripped open the snake's skin, leaving it wounded and bleeding.

The question is, whose fault was it? Was it the blind tail's fault or was it the fault of the head for giving power to its blind tail? You might find it helpful to think of your 'inner troll' as your blind tail. It might nag you into letting it take the lead, but it will ultimately lead you to self-destruction and sabotage your life force.

You Deserve More

How often have you heard someone say that they don't *deserve* something wonderful? Maybe you say it yourself – perhaps not out loud but you tend to think it. It might seem like charming modesty but actually it has serious effects. Do you remember what I told you about the unconscious mind not understanding humour? It doesn't understand subtlety or modesty either, so if you believe that you're unworthy of something, your 'inner troll' will prevent you being able to receive it.

This is the energy of poverty: we create an inner energetic poverty and programme ourselves to expect it in the future. This means that we exist in a state of constant lack. We believe that there isn't enough to go round – whether that's love or money or health, or whatever else it is that we feel we don't deserve. Maybe we believe that someone else's good fortune means we'll miss out.

Every time we feel bad about spending money (however little) on ourselves we tap into the energy of poverty. All this does is perpetuate our sense of being undeserving or unworthy. So, the next time you're broke and are worried about spending money, instead of saying 'I can't afford that,' try saying 'I choose not to buy that at the moment.' This sends a much more positive message to yourself.

The navel chakra governs whether we feel we deserve good things, so it's important to strengthen it if you're operating from a sense of lack, or the conviction that you're not entitled to good and positive things.

THE THREE ENERGY PATHOGENS

Making Yourself Small

Have you ever started a phone call by saying 'Hi, it's only me'? It seems like a perfectly ordinary thing to say, doesn't it? Especially if you have a close link with the person you're calling. However, there's a lot more going on than that. It's really your 'inner troll' speaking, and its message is clear: 'I'm not worthy', 'I'm small', 'Never mind me' and all those other self-defeating messages that diminish you.

It's easy to fix this. Try saying 'Hello, it's me' or announcing yourself by name, or anything else that seems appropriate. But stop using words and phrases that send out the message that you aren't important or worthy of attention.

Living With Second Best

Another of the ways we activate our 'inner troll' is when we make do with second best, even though we don't have to. For example, you might choose to eat off ordinary plates that you don't particular like (and which may be chipped), while keeping your nice ones for best occasions. Or you drink wine out of cheap and chunky glasses while keeping the elegant ones in the back of a cupboard. Or you eat all your meals with ugly cutlery because you think it would be a waste to get rid of it and buy something you prefer.

Maybe, whenever you open your wardrobe you see a beautiful dress or suit that you'd love to wear but don't, because you're saving it for a special occasion. Perhaps no occasion is ever quite special enough for that outfit, so you never wear it and end up giving it away because it goes out of fashion; and then you feel guilty about having 'wasted' your money on buying it in the first place. Or perhaps you watch television while sitting on a sofa that's so uncomfortable it gives you backache, but you put up with it because you think it would be wasteful to get rid of it as it has years of use left in it.

Yes, here's our 'inner troll' in action again! It's telling us that we don't honour the present as much as the future. We're devaluing the present because we don't think it's special enough. But we *need* to value it because it's the only thing we ever have. Think about it. The past has gone and the future hasn't arrived. And it never will. It can't, because it's the future.

All we have is what's happening right now, right this minute. So we need to value and honour it. If we don't embrace that, we live our lives as though they are a rehearsal for something better, something that's more worthy. Besides, as you've already learned, your middle meridian of the *present*, Sushumna, is essential for authentic living and for manifesting your best potential. It liberates you and creates a space for new energy to come into your life.

All these limiting actions mean we're micromanaging the future and never enjoying what we have around us. We all need to think about how and where we're behaving like an energetic pauper, so we can change this behaviour.

I realize that this isn't always easy, and that occasionally we have to put up with something through sheer necessity, but in so many circumstances our limiting attitudes cannot be healthily justified. They can be so ingrained as habits that we aren't even aware of them at first, or they seem like the only sensible option, given the facts.

Becoming aware of what we're doing is the first step towards changing our thoughts and attitudes, because then we can make the switch from being energetic paupers to feeling that we're living in the present, connected to the infinite source of Universal energy. If we're connected to the present, we're in a state of attracting *more* abundance. And that's when the magic happens!

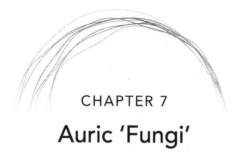

CHAPTER 7

Auric 'Fungi'

Biologically, fungi are very similar to bacteria because they both use us as their environment: they feed off us by penetrating our cells and we also share our living environment with them. Fungi are normally bigger and more complex than bacteria, yet their harmful effects are typically less severe and they develop more slowly. We're particularly prone to fungal infections when we're run-down and aren't taking good care of our nutrition or hygiene.

I expect you're wondering what auric 'fungi' could possibly be. They're the energetic equivalent of physical fungi, and they too feed off us, often in very subtle or unobtrusive ways. People who use us as their source of energy – those we commonly call 'energy vampires' – are acting very much like a fungus. They rely on our energy field to thrive.

Another example of auric fungi is stagnant energy in our living spaces, which is like a mould lurking in a corner of a room. It feeds off the energy of our arguments, dark thoughts, negative emotions and the bad vibes that we bring home.

Energy Pollution in the Home

I imagine that even if you weren't aware of the world of energy before now, you'll have noticed that different homes and buildings have different effects on you. In some places you'll feel good and light, but in others you'll feel deeply uncomfortable and heavy. Sometimes when entering a room where people have just had an argument or a conflict we say, 'You could cut the atmosphere in here with a knife.' This description demonstrates that we've picked up on the energy of the room because the conflicts and arguments have made it very dense and stagnant.

Rooms and buildings hold on to the energy that's been generated within them or released in them, whether it's positive or negative. When we meditate and are generally happy we fill our living space with positive energy, but when we argue, vent our frustration and anger about our bad day, or shout at each other, we contaminate our home with negative energy.

Just as dust and dirt can accumulate in your home if you don't clean it often enough, or you keep bringing in impurities from outside, the same thing happens at an energetic level. The fact that most of us can't see this 'energy pollution' doesn't mean it doesn't exist. It gathers in our homes like balls of physical fluff or fungus in the corner of a room.

The energy in your home has also inherited the energetic imprint of the previous owners – their personal energy and the energy of their lives. Often, without realizing it, we're moving into energetically filthy houses and flats. The previous owners may have professionally cleaned the place before you moved in but almost no one is concerned about neutralizing their energy footprints.

However, I want to emphasize something very important here, which is that all energy, in its essence, is the energy of light. It acquires negative characteristics when it becomes stagnant, heavy, and resonates at a low frequency. Our aura always tunes in to the energy of our environment, and that's especially the case with our living space. In fact, our aura often relates to our home as a part of itself, or our personal space. We live in symbiosis with our homes. Look after your home's energy and it will act as your sanctuary and protector. Your home energy also has a direct and powerful link with your base chakra. I firmly believe that this chakra is not able to function properly unless you improve your energy exchange with your living environment.

From my experience as a healer I know that sometimes just changing the energy of our living space can be enough to accelerate a very deep healing process. Also, as I described in my book *Energy Secrets*, it's important to start any healing programme or even a detox by uplifting and neutralizing our home energy. In Chapter 12, Safeguarding Barriers, you'll find advice and an exercise on cleansing the energy of the home.

Auric Fungi in Your Life

Sometimes it can be difficult to spot auric fungi, particularly when it's right under our nose. What I'm talking about here is the music we listen to, the art we enjoy, the books, magazines and newspapers we read, the films and TV programmes we watch, the podcasts we listen to, the blogs and vlogs we're signed up to, the Internet sites we return to again and again, and all the other areas of the arts and media that grab our attention every day.

We all need to exercise our awareness muscle and engage with our inner landscape, so we begin to take notice of the effect that the outer world has on us. Here's a good question to ask yourself: *What and who do I invite into my life, and am I sure I'm at peace with my choice?*

Watch What You Watch

Think about which websites you enjoy and which ones you know are bad for you. Some people feel great when they're on social media platforms while others find them a poisonous waste of time. Work out how you feel about them, so you're aware when something isn't right for you. Then you can make a *conscious* decision about whether to use them, instead of being in thrall to them and not realizing the effect they have on you.

Taking this one step further, it's important to start thinking about what you watch on TV, too. If you always watch a favourite soap opera, for instance, how do you feel afterwards? It may not be the harmless entertainment you think it is. Was it good fun and did it leave you smiling? Or did it leave you feeling anxious, annoyed or restless? Maybe you end up snapping at your partner or your children, although you're not sure why because you were fine before you watched the programme.

I'm not suggesting you should surround yourself with rosy, Pollyanna-like energy all the time, but that you need to be aware of what you're watching and the effect it has on you. You can choose to do something but it's important to reflect on the effect it will have on your internal landscape. For instance, if you're already in a sad mood, will you feel any better if you watch a tear-jerking documentary? If you're anxious, how will you feel after you've watched a gory film about a crazed mass murderer?

Some of us also need to ensure we keep our unique energy ID and don't borrow someone else's instead. There are often news stories about people who are so influenced by a particular TV programme, such as a reality show, that they over-identify with a person or character on it.

How about the music you listen to? How do you feel about some of the lyrics? Do they have positive messages for you, or do they sometimes affect you in different ways? Some of these songs may be auric fungi.

Do You Like What You See?

Now extend this to the pictures you have in your home, and even the image you choose for your computer desktop or the main page of your smartphone. Do you like what you see? Does it make you feel good? If there are paintings or photos on your walls that don't really appeal to you, or which might even make you feel slightly miserable every time you look at them, it's time to take them down and replace them with something more uplifting or neutral.

Don't worry if you can't explain *why* a particular painting or photo makes you feel bad; there may not be any obvious reason for it. However, it could be that you're picking up on the energy of the artist or photographer, or their subject matter, and it doesn't suit your particular energy frequency.

I remember once seeing an exhibition of the work of French Impressionist artist Claude Monet. I walked from room to room, loving everything I saw, until I came to some of his famous water-lily paintings. I immediately felt a depressing and oppressive energy emanating from them, and had to leave. I couldn't say why I'd felt this at the time, and it was even more inexplicable because everyone else was enjoying looking at those paintings. It was only later that I learned how unhappy and depressed Monet had been when he painted those pictures. That negative energy, which had imprinted itself on the paintings, was what I'd picked up on.

So, learn to trust your instinctive reactions to works of art, whether they're paintings, books, sculpture, music or something else. If something makes you feel uneasy, disturbed or unhappy, it's a form of auric fungi for your energy field and you need to avoid cultivating it in your environment.

Energy Vampires

Before you go to bed at night, do you always make sure you've fastened your doors and windows? Whenever you park your car, is it second nature for you to immediately lock it? But what about your aura? We know it's foolish to walk around with our handbags gaping open or our wallets sticking out of our pockets, but we may not realize that we need to lock and protect our aura too.

We aren't always aware that there are people around us who, instead of putting their hand into our purse or our bag, reach into our aura. Whenever they do this they take something much more valuable than any possession, and it's something we can't replace. Our auras are so precious!

Such people are known as 'energy vampires'. Now, as you know the word vampire usually refers to an evil creature that feeds on its human victims by sucking their blood at night. The vampire was once human itself, but after its human death it became a reanimated corpse, one of the 'living undead' as they are often called. In Russia, the word vampire originates from the Slavic *upyr* and comes from the mythology surrounding them.

But, you'll be relieved to hear, energy vampires are not the living undead. They are people who feed off the energy of others in a parasitic way. Sometimes energy vampires are attracted into our lives by the blocks we place on the mental layer of our aura – this can be, for example, when we don't feel comfortable and at ease with what we've achieved or acquired. Our guilt about this draws parasites into our lives as a way of managing our fear of abundance or success. In such cases, we'll have to work with affirmations or see a psychologist to help us to remove these mental blocks and limiting thought patterns.

How Energy Vampires Operate

Shortly, I'm going to describe some of the different ways that energy vampires can operate, but before I do that I'd like to explain how they work at an energetic or auric level. As I explained in Chapter 1, the aura has seven chakras. Five of them have two vortexes – one at the front and one at the back. However, the crown and base chakras are different. The crown chakra opens upwards and takes energy from the Universe. The base chakra opens downwards towards the ground.

As you know, the aura is formed by the collision of two forces: one from the Universe and one from the Earth. When they collide they produce the aura and this is healthy energy. We're equally nourished when we eat good food or breathe clean air.

But sometimes we become blocked and disconnected from the primal source of energy, whether as a result of psychological trauma, exhaustion, destructive emotions, illness or something else. We go into 'energy deficit' and close down the important crown and base chakras; these are meant to be positive and life-affirming but they become clogged up, like a blocked pipe.

But we still need energy, of course, so now we begin to latch onto other living beings and our environment through the other five chakras. We're no longer tapping into the abundant source of energy but pulling from the reserves of others. I'm sure you know people who are like this – when you spend time with them, you end up feeling wiped out and they walk off with a spring in their step! Sometimes we might experience that effect immediately and other times it can happen over a longer period.

Very often, people who are procrastinators – putting things off for as long as possible – or who engage in aimless tasks rather than actually doing something productive, can become energy vampires. They may appear to be busy but nothing they do has

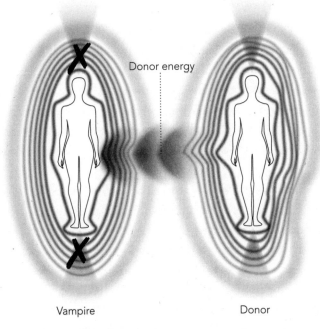

Donor energy

Vampire   Donor

Aura distortion in an energy vampire

any purpose. This creates a huge deficit in their life force, so they need to prop themselves up with other people's energy.

Some people descend to very low-frequency living and exist in the realm of their lower chakras, which are sometimes described as the realm of the animal self. They become alcoholics, drug addicts, gamblers or other types of addict. Trauma and the resulting inner void are always behind any addiction, and addicts use drugs, alcohol or other stimulants to self-regulate and to fill that void. They become energy vampires in relation to those substances.

For successful rehabilitation from addiction it's very important for the individual to focus not on the addiction itself but on filling that void with healthy energy, so they can stop repeating their behaviour. Until then, they aren't seeking an honest way to get energy – instead they are looking for donors who have high energy and will provide a quick fix (see opposite). When someone's in this state, acquiring a healthy accumulation of energy involves change; however, for some individuals this presents too much of a challenge so they find it easier to latch onto someone else.

ARE YOU AN ENERGY VAMPIRE?

Feeding off other people's energy is something we're *all* capable of doing at times: it's definitely not the case that everyone else is an energy vampire and we never are! So I'd like to invite you to reflect on where and how you feed from the energy of others in a way that drains or upsets them.

To establish whether you have a tendency towards energy vampirism, ask yourself the following questions – as with all the questions I ask you in this book, you have to be courageous enough to answer them honestly.

✧   Do people avoid making eye contact with you?

✧   Are you self-centred and believe that your opinions are facts? And do you continually need to be complimented or reassured?

✧   Are you often negative, and do you like to talk about scary scenarios and outcomes?

✧   Do you gossip about or bad-mouth people?

✧   Is it difficult for you to be alone, and do you constantly surround yourself with people or have to be in a crowd?

- ✧ Do you like to create a drama, or pick fights and arguments?

- ✧ Do you corner people and regale them with your life story or tell strangers about your misfortunes?

- ✧ Do you always ask for advice but never follow it, and do you tend to undermine other people's boundaries?

- ✧ Do you tend to induce guilt in other people and use it as way of manipulating them?

- ✧ Are you very stubborn, while expecting others to be flexible around you?

The more questions to which you answer 'yes', the more likely it is that you're an energy vampire at times. So, keep your 'third eye' on yourself and learn to acquire energy in a healthy way.

. . . .

It's also very important to ask yourself *why* you act like an energy vampire. What's your ultimate goal? When you work this out, you may be able to think of more helpful and productive ways to achieve that goal – not only for yourself but also for the people in your life. If this makes you feel uncomfortable, maybe it will help if I say again that we can *all* be energy vampires at times. But this happens less often once we start to become more aware of our behaviour.

Reserving Judgement

Be careful about who you classify as an energy vampire. Often we give the label to people who have certain psychological traits that irritate or annoy us. Sometimes we do it because someone has characteristics that we don't have but would like to. We can become energetically submissive towards this person, and deep down we resent this and put up psychological defence mechanisms that lead to energy loss.

Here's an example. Your colleague is gregarious, confident and charming; you'd love to be like him but your complexes and insecurities won't let you. This starts to irritate you because, deep down, you're aware that his energy expressions are superior to yours. Either consciously or subconsciously, you begin to envy or even hate this person. You have no reason whatsoever to develop this attitude, but you do it anyway. Now, this will create an inner conflict that will drain you of energy. Then, every time you're with this person you'll feel exhausted. This has nothing to do with your colleague being an energy vampire and everything to do with *you* detesting the fact that he has something you're striving to gain, or that you wish you possessed. Your logic and fair mind will be suppressing these unfair and negative emotions at great cost to your aura.

A similar effect is caused by people who possess qualities or a set of behaviours that we don't allow ourselves to express: perhaps those who indulge in food that we no longer permit ourselves to eat, or who live for pleasure while we're overburdened by duty. So, once again, it's important to watch your judgement. Don't assume that these people are energy vampires simply because they're having a destabilizing effect on you. They're not the ones who are draining your aura. Your irritation with them, or simply your envy, is the cause of your energy loss.

I once had a patient who always felt very drained when she was with musicians, and she concluded that musicians are energy vampires who are best avoided. It was only after a healing session with me that she recalled something from her childhood and had an 'aha' moment.

As a child she'd loved playing musical instruments and was always complimented on her talent. However, her ambitious parents became very scared that their daughter would turn into a penniless bohemian if she followed her love of music, so they steered her away from the performing arts towards science. She grew up to be a successful banker but her energy-sapping irritation with musicians was linked to her unfulfilled soul's longings and her unexpressed talents. This life-changing realization made my patient decide to take up the piano again, and she found it an incredibly healing and almost meditative experience.

We should always spend time in quiet contemplation if an irritating or draining person is mirroring our own suppressed authenticity. If you decide that this is exactly what's happening with you, you need to take proactive steps to express and harness your suppressed quality or talent. This is also why it's so important to cultivate daily gratitude for what you already have and to nourish your navel chakra, which governs the 'I love being in my skin' feeling.

What Motivates an Energy Vampire?

There are several reasons why someone becomes an energy vampire. The ideas I'm going to outline for you here draw on the work of the late Rudolf Dreikurs, an Austrian-born American psychiatrist. He adapted the work of the psychologist Alfred Adler into a practical method for understanding the difficult and challenging behaviour of children. Although Dreikurs used the following four categories to explain the reasons behind children's behaviour, I've applied them to the motives of energy vampires.

❖ **Attention-seeking behaviour:** this is the energy vampire's motivation to make others continually focus on their persona.

❖ **Power and control:** this is the tendency for the energy vampire to control everything they can. They want others to change their opinions and bend over backwards for them.

❖ **Revenge:** this applies to people who have suffered childhood trauma and are holding unresolved conflict and psychological wounds from the past. They are continually looking for ways to belittle others so they can feel better about themselves. Behind this troubling behaviour is a desire to heal psychological trauma and a sense of inferiority.

❖ **Helplessness and inadequacy:** these feelings lead to the desire to be left alone, but at the same time they make people feel they need to be helped. This person strongly believes they can't achieve what they would like to do and so they don't even try; they even hint, subtly, that they need to be rescued by others. They are defeatist and apathetic, and they want to stay in their safe little bubble.

When we engage with energy vampires and try to motivate them, we use up a huge amount of energy in our attempts to help them overcome their inertia. However, they don't shift their position. Often we even sacrifice ourselves to them until we realize much later that our help was never needed in the first place.

Help Versus Sacrifice

Here I want to emphasize something very important: help and sacrifice are not the same thing. When you help someone with the energy of your efforts and actions, without asking that person to contribute with theirs, they have no reason to change. When you sacrifice your energy you completely undermine your own boundaries and your soul's needs.

You abandon your path and start carrying the dead weight of another person's aura. This means that you become part of their dysfunctional behaviour, entering into a partnership of donor and vampire (we'll be looking at this dynamic in more detail later). Only you have the power to reverse that – they won't do it because the situation is too comfortable for them. They're getting exactly what they want. It's absolutely correct for you to expect others to take some steps towards helping themselves before you commit your energy to their cause.

I want to stress that some extreme circumstances *do* call for selfless sacrifices, but so many really don't. I trust you to exercise that judgement for yourself!

Types of Energy Vampire

There are many kinds of energy vampire, but here some of those you're most likely to come across; and don't forget that these descriptions may apply to *you* if you sometimes behave as an energy vampire.

The Emotional Blackmailer

This energy vampire is hard to spot at first, because they're so kind and so generous. Every time you see them, they'll bring you a present or buy you a treat. If you meet them for lunch or dinner, they'll insist on paying the bill, even when you've agreed to split it between you, and they probably won't even let you pay the tip. They hang on your every word and give you masses of attention, repeatedly telling you how fabulous you are.

Watch out! Although this person appears to be giving you their unconditional love, you'll gradually begin to realize that it's not unconditional at all. In fact, it's anything but. You'll feel as though you're caught in a trap because there's an invisible price tag attached to everything they're offering.

Soon, the Emotional Blackmailer will start to act in a demanding way towards you, invading your personal boundaries and treating your persona as their own. You'll want to back off from them, but you'll feel guilty every time you think about doing it because they've been so generous.

So what's really happening here? Although the Emotional Blackmailer seems to be so sincere, they've showered you with gifts and compliments in order to give themselves permission to undermine your boundaries.

They often behave in this way because of a difficult childhood. They may have grown up believing that no one will love or want them for themselves, so they need to offer incentives and rewards all the time. They may even have been abandoned as a child, and now feel unworthy of love; and they think they'll get what they're looking for if they can buy people's affection. This type of energy vampire attaches to us through the emotional layer of the aura.

The Flatterer

This energy vampire likes to penetrate your space by endlessly flattering you. They'll say things like 'I respect you so much' or 'I have a deep love for you.' Of course, it's very easy to get caught up in this trap because hearing all those compliments gives your confidence a huge boost. Who doesn't want to be told how special they are?

Unfortunately, there's a catch. These compliments are not genuine and heartfelt. When you dig deep enough, you'll discover that all this flattery is based on the Flatterer's envy of your success or happiness, or simply of the type of life you lead. They may hate you, but they want to stay in close proximity to you so they can draw energetic nourishment from you. And, unless you change the dynamic between you, that's the way it will stay.

However, if you experience personal difficulties, such as falling ill or losing a lot of money, the Flatterer will be the first person to abandon you. They'll show no remorse, either – they'll cut you out of their life and may even become your enemy, criticizing you behind your back.

An important point to remember is that this sort of energy vampire will only ever feed you with flattery and other actions that are designed to appeal to your ego. So if you ask them a question, they will always give you a flattering response. A true friend, when asked, will give you their honest opinion, even if it isn't what you want to hear.

The Manipulator

Here's another vampire who can be incredibly charming and charismatic, and they are very compassionate and attentive, too. The Manipulator will tell you they care about you, and they're always looking for ways to be useful. If you need a lift, you only have to ask. If you're having a bad time, they'll dash round with something to cheer you up.

But then they'll become too involved in your life. They'll start to take over, looking for problems and telling you what to do about them. For instance, the Manipulator can be the over-involved mother who becomes so caught up in her children's lives that she tries to control their relationships by sowing seeds of doubt about their partners. It can also be the friend who appears to be so caring and helpful, but who really wants to create drama in your life by making you suspicious about your partner's motives or fidelity.

The Manipulator can even be your boss – playing the game of being awestruck by your talents and always telling you how fantastic you are, and then getting you to do lots of extra work for them. They'll wear the mask of someone who appreciates and values your qualities, but uses compliments and praise to manipulate you into giving them your energy. This vampire can be quite ruthless in the way they operate.

The Green-Eyed Monster

This is someone who desperately wishes they were as happy, positive and healthy as you are. They'll judge you harshly if you possess any of the radiant qualities that they would like to have; and they'll make you feel bad about them – perhaps with comments that seem OK on the surface, but which, on closer analysis, contain barbs. It's a form of jealousy; the Green-Eyed Monster feels they're failing to be the person they'd like to be, so they'll do their best to bring you down to their level, rather than rise to meet yours.

Often, this is the person who'll ply you with alcohol to make you drunk, even when you tell them you aren't drinking, or make you stay up late, despite knowing that you like to go to bed early. Once you've regressed to their level it will give them an energy boost.

The Paranoid Vampire

This person is oversensitive and loves to produce a drama out of nothing. In Russia, we call it creating an elephant out of a fly! They always detect a hidden, and negative, meaning in everything that happens, and always take it personally, convinced that it's directed at them. They can't trust anyone and believe that we all have an agenda.

The Paranoid Vampire is incredibly rigid; if others don't abide by *their* code of behaviour, they become very upset and wary. If you make a mistake and apologize for it, the Paranoid Vampire will never forget it, and they'll always manage to remind you of it. If you upset them, they'll never trust you again.

They'll even twist reality to support their idea of what you're *really* like, and will find a way to manipulate situations so they can justify their negative and paranoid opinion of you. It's exhausting to be on the receiving end of the Paranoid Vampire's behaviour because they'll make you doubt yourself and mistrust your own energy space. And that, of course, is exactly what they want as they'll feed off your disturbed energy.

The Fair-Weather Vampire

If you're going through a good phase or have something to celebrate, the Fair-Weather Vampire will be right by your side. You'll have the impression that they really like you and enjoy your company, and you'll like being with them, too. But, at the first sign of trouble – when you hit a difficult emotional phase, perhaps, or become unwell – they'll disappear. They won't get in touch, they won't return your calls, and your emails will seemingly have vanished into a big black hole.

You can enjoy being with this person but don't expect them to be something they aren't; and don't invest in them at a deep level, because they'll never meet you there. You'll only end up being used as a prop for their emotional energy.

The Peacock

The ego has landed! Peacocks are completely wrapped up in themselves. They can't stop showing off to you about their achievements and letting you know how incredible they are. Networking is second nature to them – and often done in quite a ruthless way – and they could easily make use of your contacts, too. Eventually, you'll realize that they are simply using you as a mirror in which they can admire their own reflection.

They aren't interested in you – they're only interested in your admiration of them or in having you as their backdrop. Once you begin to see this, you'll realize that the conversation is rarely, if ever, about you: it's about them; and even if they come across as full of empathy and warmth, you'll soon discover that this is a ploy to engage your energy and use you as a prop for their massive ego. The only thing the Peacock wants to hear you say is how fabulous they are. It's as though you don't really exist, other than as a reflection of them.

Smother Love

This vampire–donor dynamic is normally played out between a mother and her child. As we explored earlier, a mother's base chakra is connected to her baby's base chakra, but when the umbilical cord is cut after birth the mother is still connected to her baby through an energetic cord that runs between their navel chakras.

This energetic connection lasts between nine and 10 years, and then the child starts to become independent and energetically separate. However, if the mother has gone through some sort of trauma that has made her needy, possessive and controlling, she won't allow this separation to take place. Instead, she'll swamp her child with a suffocating form of love.

This also happens if the mother is longing for companionship but doesn't find it, because her partner is 'unavailable', perhaps, or because she's single. As a result, she never gets a chance to find a new partner, and the child, too, doesn't form the personal space in which to develop a successful romantic partnership or healthy friendships. Even as an adult that child will feel as if they're always sharing their mother's energy field. This impediment to the formation of their personal space will also lead to a lack of immunity to the toxic energies in their life.

The Temporary Energy Vampire

Sometimes, being an energy vampire is only a temporary state. One of the most common ways for this to happen is when someone is ill. They start to feel sorry for themselves – moaning or making a big fuss about how unwell they feel – and when you ask them how they are they'll exaggerate their symptoms to get your sympathy. I suspect we've all been guilty of doing this from time to time, but we don't continue in this state once we start to feel better.

Full-On Chatterbox

This is the person who never stops talking. They chat away about anything and everything, but it's not a conversation because they aren't talking *to* you, they're talking *at* you. They ignore the fact that you're only listening out of politeness, and they talk at length about people you've never met, even showing you endless photos of them. Unsurprisingly, you soon become drained by this.

Whenever the Full-On Chatterbox calls you, you don't know how to end the conversation because they keep thinking of new things to say. If you meet them in the street, you feel trapped and don't know how to get away from them. Sometimes this is a friend who goes through a never-ending string of dramas, so there's always something that dominates their conversation and demands everyone's attention.

Grey Mouse

When you first meet a Grey Mouse you never imagine that this meek and mild person is an energy vampire. They speak so softly and quietly that you have to strain your ears to hear them, and *that's* how they get your attention. Once they have it, you begin to realize that they're always melancholy, and there's always something wrong.

You'll never see a Grey Mouse laughing hard or smiling sincerely because they're far too miserable for that. And soon, you'll feel equally miserable when you're with them, as you begin to resonate with their frequency and attune to their wavelength, all of which comes when you adjust your hearing to the quietness of their voice.

The Firework

Stand well back! Whenever you're around this person it's like walking a tightrope because they could lose their temper at any moment. They're so fiery and short-tempered, and so quick to ignite, that you feel scared when you're with them and make yourself smaller inside so you won't provoke them.

The Firework is also prone to competitiveness, and they don't want anyone else to be a winner. It's a sign that they feel superior to everyone else. This person will always choose war over peace, both in actions and words. They like to create conflict and will always believe they're in the right and everyone else is wrong or guilty. If they have a complaint, they'll want to take it to the highest authority. They look for ways to reduce you – their opponent – to nothing because they want to belittle you. They get their fix when you're out of your comfort zone, reacting fearfully and being energetically submissive.

The Bully

This type of energy vampire is very similar to the Firework in that they want to belittle you, but the Bully does it by pressing your buttons. They like to single out a person, often because they are different in some way, and then be cruel to them, picking up on their insecurities or physical imperfections. The person who is being bullied will keep reacting, which is what gives the Bully their energy fix. Someone who is energetically strong will never rely on another person for their fix – which means the Bully is, by definition, an energetically weak person.

Look But Don't Touch

Here's someone whose appearance and way of dressing is always provocative, whether it's short skirts and low-cut tops, very low-slung jeans, bright colours, lots of piercings, a whole library of tattoos or masses of make-up. They do this because they want to feed off your attention, and they're always looking for your reaction, whether it's good or bad.

Often, this person likes to provoke in another way too: with overtly sexual behaviour and language; yet they remain unavailable, so they feed off the energy of other people's desires. They use their sexual energy as a bait to capture your interest, but it ends up almost possessing you and keeps you dangling on their hook. Look But Don't Touch can be very young, incredibly beautiful or handsome, and sexy, and they give you a very small amount in return for taking a lot.

In Part 5 of the book I'll teach you various techniques for managing energy vampires and ways to curb your own tendencies to energy vampirism.

Part IV

. . . .

A
DIS-EASE
OF THE
21ST CENTURY

CHAPTER 8

The Digital Layer of the Aura

The ideas I'm proposing in this section of the book may startle you, but they're something I feel passionately about. As I explained in Chapter 1, traditionally there are seven layers of the human aura; I described the first three in detail because they're the layers that are most involved in everything I've written about in this book. However, to my surprise, I'm beginning to realize that in the Western world of the 21st century, people are developing an eighth layer in the aura. It's a *digital* layer.

Our aura had to metamorphose in order to adapt to the changes in our environment. And, unlike most evolutionary changes, the digital revolution happened incredibly quickly, so we have to consciously help our body and aura to find harmony with this newly emerged reality.

Our Digital Environment

Today, our lives are slowly being taken over by digital technology: it's hard to find a home that doesn't have multiple screens, Wi-Fi and all manner of electronic gadgets. They've almost become a part of the family. Mobile phones have shrunk dramatically since they first appeared in the 1980s, so now we can carry them around in a pocket. Our computers are immensely faster and more efficient than they used to be, and if we wish to, we can have a computerized system in the corner of a room that will provide an answer whenever we ask it a question, or even order food for us.

The Internet has revolutionized our lives in ways we could only have imagined a few years ago, from online banking to live streaming of music and movies, and from instant information to the ability to see and chat with someone in a different time zone on the other side of the world. The almost universal use of the Internet has also given birth to our online personas. We project our presence into cyberspace through our various accounts and profiles, and many of us have begun to exist in a virtual life alongside our real one. And our online persona is beginning to echo back at us.

For example, let's say you're starting to relate to one of your social media accounts as an extension of yourself. The avatars and names you initially created as a mask are now 'eating' into your true face. These kinds of crossovers, and the fact that digital devices constantly inhabit our aura, have created a new current of energy in our aura – the digital layer.

I don't necessarily regard this as a pathology, but more as our way of adapting to a change in our environment. However, the reason I've written this chapter is because this digital layer is increasingly starting to act in a dominant, all-consuming way. It's slowly taking over our energy ID by manipulating our relationship with the Self and the real world.

We're increasingly relying on our computers for even minor mental tasks, which is leading the digital energy to intertwine with the mental layer of our aura. A lot of our emotional energy is becoming reliant on the boost we get whenever others engage in our social media posts or 'like' our uploaded photographs. We're adapting our inner flow to the rapid speed of our digital devices.

By looking to our computers for grounding and inspiration we're disconnecting from our primal sources of energy: terrestrial and Universal. We're starting to align with the digital stream instead of the flow of nature's energies and, as a result, this new surrogate energy source is producing a new kind of aura. So, I believe that now is the time for us to redress the balance.

In only a few years, digital technology has altered our lives beyond recognition; but for many of us, it's starting to dominate. We take our devices to the dinner table and engage with them instead of each other. We take our devices to bed, so we can catch up on the latest conversation on social media before switching off the light.

We might even check them again when we wake in the middle of the night, or reach for them first thing in the morning before we've even got out of bed. When we're out and about, we clutch hold of our smartphones or tuck them into a pocket so we can grab them as soon as they ring or send us an alert. It's not too far-fetched to say that some people now view their smartphones as an extension of themselves.

Most people wouldn't want any of this to change, and I think in many ways digital devices are of enormous benefit to us. However the digital environment is becoming like a puppet master, and instead of our devices serving us, they are increasingly turning people into their puppets. I'm already seeing plenty of patients who are suffering from digital overload and are desperate to wean themselves off their reliance on their devices.

Our digital devices are becoming our energy vampires! We're often at their mercy, and their bleep is our command. We jump whenever they start flashing or make a sound. Our devices take our energy and we willingly surrender our boundaries to them. We give up our personal space in return for instant gratification and validation through social media 'likes'.

Digital Pollution

Our phones, computers, tablets, laptops, routers, smart TVs and even the little fitness gadgets we wear on our wrists use electromagnetic waves to transmit data and signals. And as we explored earlier, the natural world, including your body, produces electromagnetic fields and our aura is also electromagnetic in nature.

But these natural fields are low in intensity. Modern technology produces much more intense electromagnetic fields and these can lead to health risks. Strong artificial electromagnetic fields can interfere with your aura and the natural way your body works. So, when dealing with our digital devices, our awareness should not only be on the aura-altering effects of the Internet but also on its toxic electromagnetic radiation.

You're familiar by now with my insights into the way we synchronize with our neighbouring energy fields, and I'm afraid we tend to display a very similar synchronization with our digital devices. Just as you adjust your pace when walking with a friend, you adjust your inner energy rhythms when you're with your devices. And as you're about to find out, this alters your interaction with light. All of this is happening so fast in evolutionary terms that our aura and body are struggling to adapt in a healthy way. It makes me, as a healer, so sad to see people's energy owned by their devices. This will never lead to an authentic and fulfilling life or a healthy body.

Ring, Ring

What do you do with your mobile phone at night? Do you switch it off? Do you leave it in a bag or on a table? Is it in your bedroom or in another room? Do you put it on your bedside table, so you can check your emails or update your social media accounts just before you go to sleep, and so its alarm setting can wake you up in the morning? Or maybe you keep it under your pillow, so you can grab it whenever you need it?

Although it might be convenient to keep your phone close to you, there are many reasons why this isn't such a good idea. A series of experiments has found that having a mobile phone close to your head (which it will be if it's on your bedside table or nestling beneath your pillow) changes the pattern of activity in the regions of your brain that are nearest the phone.

Your brain's basic 'resting' behaviour is affected by this.[1,2] It isn't yet known what the long-term effects might be, but we do know that our brainwaves change when a mobile phone is actively sending and receiving signals. The current assumption is that these effects will be slow, gradual changes in our mental presence and alertness.[3]

As a healer, however, I can say that your phone causes a huge interference in your third eye and crown chakras, which are the two important chakras for intuition and recharging. This contributes to the lack of ability many of us have to access our intuition or attune with the Universe.

How Do You Sleep?

Normally, our body and brain keep track of time, including whether it's day or night, based on light levels and changes in our hormone levels. This happens automatically, like so many other functions that are controlled by our brain. When we lie in a bed in a darkened room and relax, our brain realizes what we're doing and our brainwaves shift into a pattern that's designed to send us off to sleep.

Alarmingly, however, the electronics that have become such an integral part of our homes can disrupt these sleep schedules, preventing our body from synchronizing with regular day–night cycles. Instead of effortlessly slipping into sleep as our brainwaves shift into a sleep-inducing pattern, we can take ages to drop off and may not manage it at all. This is because the radiation emitted by phone signals and radio waves disrupts the brain's natural patterns of electrical activity.[4,5] In other words, our brain synchronizes with these radiation signals and this can literally keep us awake at night.

Even more concerning is new evidence suggesting that the constant broadcast of radio and phone signals not only affects our ability to fall asleep, it affects us all night long, shifting our sleeping habits and increasing the amount of REM (rapid eye movement) sleep we get.[6,7] It's when we're in the REM phase that we dream most vividly, so you might imagine that this isn't such a problem. Vivid dreams can be really entertaining.

However, if we spend too long in the REM phase of sleep each night, we don't get enough of the other stages of sleep (light sleep and deep sleep). It's during these light- and deep-sleep stages that we're able to relax; our breathing and heart rate become regular, our body recovers from our daily exertions, vital hormones are discharged to balance the stress hormones released during the day, and the body carries out any muscle repairs that are necessary.

It's not only radios and mobile phones that can affect our ability to get a good night's sleep. Wi-Fi routers do it, too. Our brains synchronize with their radiation, which affects the body's basic rhythms in two worrying ways. The first is, once again, our sleep patterns. Wi-Fi can contribute to insomnia: as the ultra-fast pulses of radiation sent out by the router hit our body and brain, they may be disrupting the electrical signals the body uses to control sleep, thereby keeping us awake; and, when we do get to sleep, they make that sleep less restful.[8]

You might be wondering what's wrong with that – after all, we all have restless nights every now and then yet we usually manage to recover. That's true, but we can't recover if it happens to us every time we go to sleep. The second way that Wi-Fi is known to affect us is by reducing our mental function, probably also because the brain isn't synchronizing with the signals it sends out.[9]

So here's a suggestion. The next time you can't sleep, try turning off your router or modem for the night. Not only will it let your brain return to its regular, healthy rhythms, it might help stop you checking your email or social media accounts in the early hours of the morning.

Smartphones and other devices, including televisions, can also affect our ability to fall asleep because of the blue light they emit. This light reduces the amount of melatonin the brain produces, and that's important because it's melatonin that regulates our circadian rhythms and therefore our ability to fall asleep.[10] Spending too much time online late at night, or even up to three hours before going to sleep, can trick our brain into thinking it's still daytime and that therefore we aren't yet ready for sleep. This means that our brain has synchronized with the blue light being emitted by our devices.

Staying in Control

As I've just explained, science is showing that we tend to synchronize with our devices in ways that are similar to the ways we synchronize with other people. For most of us, though, giving up digital technology isn't a realistic possibility, and nor do I call for it. However, if we want to seek balance and an authentic flow in our lives, we mustn't *ignore* this new digital layer. This means we must harness our online personas and be the master whenever we interact with our devices. In other words, we must make sure that *we're* the ones in control, not them.

The frequencies at which digital gadgets and electronics work are so much faster than our human frequencies, which is why so many of us are feeling that we're constantly trying to catch up with our devices. Our personal space is being continually invaded by the alerts, sounds and displays that our smartphones, computers, tablets and other gadgets emit all day long – and, sometimes, all night too.

Some of us are able to manage this electronic onslaught to some extent – by switching off our devices at times, or at least muting their sound – but that isn't the case for everyone. Studies have shown that there's a correlation between certain personality types and an inability to create boundaries with electronic devices. It seems that anyone with an addictive personality, or who is a people-pleaser, or is shy, lonely or has low self-esteem, tends to be affected much more strongly by this constant demand for their attention than those who are non-addictive and confident.[11,12]

I can add that in my healing practice I've noticed that people with depleted auras or blocked base and navel chakras tend to attach themselves to their devices more than anyone else. It has become their surrogate way of grounding, creating a connection to their tribe of people, and their source of validation. Our online life is starting to act like a sticking plaster for our depleted natural life force.

Are You Addicted to Your Phone?

Scientists and other researchers have been studying the addictive nature of mobile phone usage since 2005. It's clear that using a mobile or smartphone can be addictive because of the way that some of us let them rule our lives.[13,14] If you're wondering whether this applies to you, take a look at some of these indications that you may be addicted to your phone:

1. You feel compelled to use your phone all the time.

2. The moment you hear the ping of a social media alert or an email landing in your inbox, you immediately feel compelled to see what it is, and you feel anxious if you can't do that for some reason.

3. You clutch your phone in your hand almost all the time, reluctant to put it down.

4. You continually check your phone, even when having a face-to-face conversation with someone, when you're eating, out walking the dog, and possibly even when you're in a cinema or theatre.

5. You take your phone into the loo with you, in case you get an alert or email that you need to read.

6. Friends and loved ones complain they can never get your full attention because you're so easily distracted by your phone.

7. You sleep with your phone next to you, so you can check it whenever you wake during the night.

8. The way you use your phone is significantly disrupting your life.

It's also recognized that the percentage of time that someone spends specifically on social-networking applications is a strong predictor of whether they'll become addicted to their phones. Another indicator is the size and density of someone's online network. In other words, the more social media sites you use and the more friends and followers you have on them, the more likely you are to become addicted to them.

If you use your phone purely as a camera, you aren't addicted to it. Of course, it's a different story if you regularly post the photos you take with it all over social media or are continually emailing them to your friends.

In the next chapter, I'm going to show you how to manage the digital layer of your aura.

CHAPTER 9

Digital Living Versus Digital Slavery

Most of us have no choice but to welcome the digital technology that has transformed our lives over the past few decades. It's here to stay. Even so, I believe that we all need to balance our digital life with our real life. Instead of going into a state of denial about the way technology has changed things and saying that all electronic devices are bad and must be avoided, I believe that we must embrace them on our own terms, and from the perspective of our authentic self.

However, I do think it's crucial that we all try to resist an all-consuming digital saturation that will wipe out our boundaries and our personal space, and hijack our inner rhythms, such as our 'body clock'. Each of us needs to ensure we boost our metabolism so it's strong enough to resist the incredibly rapid pace of digital technology.

Digital Layer Dominance

As I explained in the previous chapter, we're beginning to develop a digital layer in our aura, but we must not allow it to run us as if we're a computer program. Humans create tools that we can use. We can't allow those tools to use *us*, which is what happens when the digital layer takes over.

In fact, it's always dangerous when *any* of the layers of the aura start to dominate, because it's not a balanced situation. When the mental layer takes over we become too cerebral. When the emotional layer does so, we become completely immersed in our emotions and lose our sense of self. And when our physical layer dominates, we become very primitive when dealing with relationships and life, and we lose our emotional intelligence.

In other words, if any layer of the aura becomes dominant, we lose our Self and disrupt our unique frequency. The new digital layer is infiltrating us, like a digital virus on our phone or computer. Digital technology was developed to make our lives easier but now it rules them. Where does it end?

Many of us are controlled by our phone alerts and updates. We're developing a compulsive relationship with all those beeps and buzzes and vibrations, to the degree that our inner state is becoming dependent on our devices. It's so important for us that we don't become disconnected from real life because we're so wrapped up in the electronic world instead.

Own Your Angle of Perception

When I visit art galleries I often notice that the people around me aren't looking directly at the paintings and sketches on the walls because they're too busy snapping photos of them with their phones, or taking selfies. I notice the same thing at school sports days and children's end-of-term concerts. Lots of the spectators aren't actually watching what's going on, they're filming it instead, so they can watch it later.

Of course, from my perspective as a healer, this sort of behaviour takes us away from our central meridian of now and sways us towards the meridian of the future. This causes a distortion of our life force and is a huge waste of the precious energy of the present moment.

Anyone who views their life through the screen of their phone receives a very narrow picture of it. They're denied the chance to choose what they're looking at because when we look at a screen we're seeing *someone else's* angle of perception. We can't see what's happening outside the angle of the screen. We all have to protect our *own* angle and the way we perceive the world around us. We have to see it for ourselves and not in the way that our device chooses to show it to us.

Securing our personal space and protecting our energy cannot be separated from protecting our inner space and maintaining our own angle of perception. Personally, I find it very alarming to see the degree to which we're synchronizing with the much faster pace of the digital age. We don't own our moments if we're always checking our screens and instantly reacting to what we see on them. And if we don't own our moments we can't own our energy. We've given it away to someone or something else, and now it's calling the shots.

Our Energy in the 'Digital Village'

Before the advent of the digital revolution, it was relatively easy for us to keep our public and private lives separate. But now that we live in a 'digital village' so many of our personal boundaries have been blurred or removed.

Many of us are now over-sharing in our public and private lives, and as a result we're becoming overexposed. Personal data that most of us would never have shared with others in the past is now common currency. We broadcast information about our lives to everyone – we aren't selective about it at all. We even use apps on our phones that announce on social media where we've been or where we are in the present moment.

Allowing another person into our lives is an intimate process, and it takes time to build up a relationship. So, in the same way that we don't invite everyone into our home, we should be selective about who we invite into our virtual lives. Many of us share all our personal information in order to create online friendships, but often it's not done in a healthy way. I think it's almost a form of exhibitionism – designed to get 'likes' from others, to win their sympathy when things go wrong, or their admiration when we've something to boast about.

This sort of personal validation might give us an initial boost, but it's a short-lived surrogate with illusionary effects. What's more, it's addictive, because that validation will be fleeting and we'll soon need more of it. So we'll post something else that's very personal in the hope of attracting more 'likes'. If this continues, our sense of self-worth and our happiness become overly dependent on other people's approval and attention, and that affects our energy. We feel good when we get positive responses from a group of virtual friends and bad when we don't. Is this a healthy situation? No!

We might be part of a virtual tribe yet we're more disconnected from one another physically, emotionally and mentally than ever before. At the very least, social media platforms collect, store and use our personal data. We need to be mindful of that. Think about it: if you kept a diary, would you want it to be stored somewhere by strangers so they could refer to it whenever they wanted to find out something about you or try to sell you a product? Your unique energy ID is up for sale, so you can be flooded with advertising waves calibrated to match your frequency.

Digital Immigrants and Digital Natives

Are we all slaves to the Internet? Members of the older generation, who are often referred to as 'digital immigrants', would probably answer with a resounding 'yes'. They are the people who generally find it easiest to resist the seductive and addictive nature of the digital age because they can recall the time before it existed. They can remember when, instead of emailing or texting each other, we sent letters and postcards or we picked up the phone and arranged to meet friends socially.

Younger people, and especially millennials, who are sometimes called 'digital natives', tend to struggle a lot more when trying to avoid becoming completely immersed in digital life. That's because they grew up surrounded by digital gadgets and technology and don't have a personal non-digital point of reference. There are even signs that some younger people experience reality as something that happens on-screen, rather than in person. They may only relate to the world through their devices, or they may interact with people's avatars rather than through direct human-to-human contact.

Flawed Humans?

Although this may seem a bizarre concept, the content and design of many technological devices and online programs stems from the assumption that human beings are flawed. (And especially so when we're compared to computers.) I find this alarming. However, it's an unavoidable fact that we're starting to rely on computers and the Internet so much that we're thinking for ourselves less and less often.

For example, when we're looking for something online, many of us click on the first couple of Web pages that come up in our search results and never think to investigate any of the others. And when we're calculating a figure, many of us reach for the calculators on our phones rather than doing some quick mental arithmetic – something that was second nature to previous generations.

Above all, we're starting to trust our computers more than our own intuition. This is really dangerous because our intuition is the ultimate tool for refining our unique energy ID. If we don't have this, because we've handed over all control to our devices, there will be no room for authentic humans – only for generic beings. What's more, computer programs are created by humans, so handing over our unique energy ID to them means we're allowing ourselves to be programmed, just like robots, by someone else's ideas of what we should be doing and thinking.

We humans have evolved through countless generations to exist in a world with its own speed and pace. Our fulfilment and our experience of our true self is very much linked to the natural environment. Yes, machines can sometimes operate faster than any human, but we'll lose our authentic life if everything in it is delegated to our devices.

Living an Artisanal Life

The good news is that it doesn't have to be like this. Consider for a minute the difference between the creations produced by artisans and the items mass-produced in factories. The artisan's work has individuality, because they will have put something of their own personality into it, and every piece they craft will be slightly different, whereas mass-produced articles are identical.

So, I'm encouraging you to be like an artisan, but an artisan *creating your own unique life.* Yes, you can delegate some things to your devices, but not everything. And don't allow yourself to be moulded by the suggestive projected images on the Internet. It's OK to be challenged and to have to think things through, to process the information and refine your tactics by yourself. You don't have to rely on an algorithm to give you – and everyone else – its own set of answers or guidance for living. And especially not when that algorithm is designed to sell you something, make you press a series of 'click-bait' links, or capture masses of your personal data.

Throughout history we humans have made our own tools and used them. I don't want the situation to be reversed, so our tools start using us and become our masters! Our devices should create opportunities for us, rather than turn us into passive observers who are unconsciously manipulated by whatever it is that we find online.

The Manipulation of Time

So far I've been talking about the way our digital devices are affecting our relationship with our Self, our environment and the state of our aura. But according to some psychologists, technology is having a profound effect on how we're experiencing the passing of time, too.

Of course, time is a subjective experience. As I'm sure you know only too well, five minutes can disappear in a flash when you're dashing around first thing in the morning, frantically trying to get ready for the day ahead. But those five minutes can feel more like five very long hours when you're sitting nervously in the dentist's chair, having a tooth filled!

Have you ever wondered what gives us our sense of time? Scientists have made the fascinating discovery that the human brain contains an internal clock that governs our perception of how fast time is passing, depending on our circumstances. They know that neurotransmitters in the brain, including dopamine and norepinephrine, play a vital role in our perception of time, although science still can't explain exactly how this works.

Putting it simply, whenever we experience something, our brain is able to gather the information and process it, but not necessarily in the order in which we received it. We quickly process information that we're already familiar with, but when we're confronted with something new it takes more time for our brain to assimilate and process every piece of that information, which is why time then seems to slow down. That's why a journey that we've never taken before can feel longer than it does once we know the way.

The amount of attention we pay to a particular task also affects our perception of the passing of time, so an unfamiliar task seems to take longer because we're noticing what we're doing. When we're familiar with that task, it seems to take less time to complete.

However, our perception of time is now being altered in a new way. Constant access to virtually unlimited amounts of news and updates can create a need for immediacy that speeds up both our intake of information and our perception of time. Technology makes us impatient with anything that takes more than a few seconds to achieve, as you'll know if you've ever started to scroll through a blog or news article, not found what you wanted immediately, and clicked off it again in frustration.

The hyper-connectivity of the Internet age can contribute to a need for instant gratification and a lack of patience. We want it now and we aren't prepared to wait! Sadly, this leads to an inability to focus on the bigger picture of our true needs and simply traps us in a cycle of quick fixes and instant gratification.

In this digital era, the energy of the present moment is constantly being disrupted and devalued. The flow in the Sushumna meridian of now is constantly being sabotaged and overtaken by channels of past and future by this very modern tendency. However, as I've already mentioned, your ability to own your energy is very much linked to your ability to connect to the present moment.

Connecting to the Present Moment

Are you hoping to enjoy a long life? I think most of us are. Would you like to know the secret of achieving it? If we can protect the energy of the present moment – the moment right here, right now – we'll live longer; or perhaps more precisely we'll *feel alive* for longer. Yes, biologically, the number of years we live may remain the same but we'll experience them as lasting for a much longer period. The majority of us are focusing on extending the length of our life but I want to help you to restore a healthier time perception so your life seems fuller as well as longer.

Practising mindfulness can help us connect to the present moment and make our lives feel more satisfying. Mindfulness has many benefits, including increasing our attention span and improving our memory. It also slows down our perception of time because it enables us to engage fully with each moment instead of letting it pass us by while we're distracted by something else.[1]

Train yourself to pay attention to the details of whatever it is you're doing, and to keep a sense of wonder rather than taking reality for granted. The more you're anchored in and appreciative of your real life, the less willing you'll be to sacrifice your life force on the altar of digital living. Often we give ourselves, and our life, away because of a lack of awareness and self-reflection. We just go with the digital flow towards a short 'fully alive time'.

Mindfulness must be introduced into our lives alongside a much healthier relationship with our electronic devices. Both will help us to protect our 'internal metronome of time'.

Keeping Our Digital Aura in Balance

By now you may be wondering how you can manage the digital layer of your aura, if it's here to stay. As I've already said, I'm not suggesting we all give away our electronic devices and renounce this new digital era, but there are important steps we can all take to protect ourselves and keep our aura in balance.

The Digital Detox

A lot is said these days about the importance of having regular digital 'detoxes'. Perhaps you already know about these – but do you actually do them? If you're new to the idea, it simply means switching off your digital devices for a set amount of time each day or week and doing something instead that isn't reliant on information technology or electronic devices.

That could be anything you like. How about chatting to a friend, talking to your partner, listening as your child tells you about their day, going for a relaxing walk, watching the birds in your garden, or curling up with a favourite book?

Start Small

If you've never given yourself a digital detox before, or the thought of being disconnected from your phone or tablet makes you feel slightly panicky, you need to start small. Decide that for just 10 minutes each day – or half an hour, if you can manage it – you're going to switch off every digital device in your home and do something peaceful for yourself. Make this a habit.

Be aware though that it's not enough simply to switch off the *sound* on your phone or computer. Experiments have found that we can still be distracted by our device when it's quiet, especially if we're sitting close to it. You'll find it easier to focus on what you're doing if your phone or device is in another room, so you can forget about it for the time being.[2]

Keep Your Distance

It can also help to put your phone in airplane mode whenever you aren't using it. This will stop it pinging with alerts all the time, and it will also reduce the amount of radiation it's emitting. You can switch it back to its normal mode whenever you want to use it.

I see a lot of people carrying their phones in a pocket, so that it's next to their body, or in their hand. This might be convenient for them, especially if they're expecting an important call or text, but it increases their exposure to the electromagnetic fields emitted by their phone and multiplies the chances of aura contamination. It's much better to carry our phone away from our body. When we want to talk on the phone, we should use earpieces and not hold the device next to our head.

Many of us own laptops or tablets, too, and when using these we should keep them away from our body as much as possible – again, to reduce our exposure to their electromagnetic fields. Instead of balancing your laptop on your knees, which means that toxic EMF emissions will go through your body, try to remember to put it on a table or on a special electromagnetic field blocking pad that will deflect harmful waves away from your body.

Banish Your Phone from the Bedroom

Another very important step is to keep your phone out of your bedroom at night. If you normally leave it switched on, maybe on your bedside table, when you go to sleep, you need to turn it off and leave it in another room. Please note: you have to do *both* of these things.

Even if you decide to have your phone in your bedroom at night, don't keep it by your bedside with the sound on so you can hear the arrival of every email or social media alert. Turn off the sound, so your sleep (and/or your partner's) isn't continually disturbed by an endless series of beeps. These audio signals are particularly disruptive to our energy when we're asleep and our natural defences are down. They cause our energy to flow in a chaotic manner because they disrupt our unique frequency.

Being Available in the Digital Age

Something else to be aware of these days is the amount of time you spend being available to others. It can add up to many more hours than you think. Consider carefully how much time you spend online, and how often you check your phone or email each day. Of course, you need to be realistic and honest about this, because if you just make a guess, it's almost guaranteed to be less than the true figure.

You must also make sure that you don't get caught up in the idea that you *have* to respond instantly to emails, social media alerts, text messages and phone calls. Just because you have access to a phone or computer, it doesn't mean you have to be constantly available.

Although this sounds rather ironic, we can download useful apps to help us monitor the amount of time we spend on our smartphones and tablets. I suggest that you investigate these apps so you can monitor your daily usage. Some will track the amount of time you spend on social media sites and others will record the number of times you check your phone in a day. Apps like these, which are being developed all the time, are useful because the information they provide can be quite eye-opening. For instance, even though you imagine that you only spend an hour a day scrolling through social media sites on your phone, you might discover that it's much more than that.

Setting Digital Boundaries

It's really important that you give yourself permission to adapt to the digital age at your own pace and in your own way. Sometimes you may have to respond to an email or text immediately, of course, but that doesn't mean you must always jump to attention the minute your phone or computer sounds an alert. If you put yourself in the position of responding as soon as an email lands in your inbox or a text appears, you'll create a rushed pace throughout your day.

What's more, you'll be allowing other people to set that pace and to dictate what you do with your day. That doesn't leave any room for your authentic existence and you'll end up behaving like a puppet. This might sound extreme to you but if you're always checking your phone or interrupting what you're doing to reply to texts or emails the minute they arrive, you really are allowing other people to rule your life. They're pulling the strings and you're doing the dancing.

Of course, we all have to be flexible about when it's appropriate to respond immediately and when it isn't, but we also need to use the power of self-reflection. Decide which digital strings are pulling on you and then prioritize them, just like any other hierarchy of values. You may decide that other things in your life are more important than these digital strings.

Instead of continually checking your emails, maybe you could sign out of your email account, so you aren't tempted to take a sneaky peek at it, and only check it once an hour. Or maybe once every two hours, depending on the circumstances. Once you get used to doing this, you may be able to allow longer gaps between checking your emails and texts. You can do the same with the social media sites you belong to. You might even decide to turn off their constant notifications of new messages and postings, so you're no longer distracted by them throughout the day.

Are you honestly interested in most of them anyway, or are they just a momentary distraction from what you're meant to be doing? Instead of staring at a screen, maybe you could talk to the people around you, or do something else that you enjoy!

Time Your Online Activity

When you do visit a social media site or want to play an online game, decide in advance how long you're going to spend on it and then set an alarm, so you know when your time is up. If you don't do this, you may find that you've been sucked into the site and have lost all sense of time passing, and then you'll feel guilty or annoyed with yourself for wasting time. Remember, social media and online games sites might be financially free but you're still paying for them with your precious life force and priceless present moments.

The media often talks about the number of children who spend hours online each day, but there are also growing numbers of kids who complain about their parents' addiction to their phones or computers. The parents aren't available for their children because their attention is being hijacked by digital technology. If parents want to have a good relationship with their children they must be very careful about their own use of technology, so that it doesn't take over their lives.

I run retreats at many top spas, and they don't allow their guests to use computers or phones during their stay. In the pre-digital past, spas didn't allow smoking, but now they insist on being technology-free zones too. But you don't need to stay in a spa to set up your own digital-free zone. Do it daily, or even weekly, and make sure you don't combine your virtual and real lives. Focus on one or the other, rather than both at the same time. This means you can be fully engaged with what you're doing, rather than continually distracted.

More Tools for Reclaiming Your Energy

Here are some other ideas for balancing both your real and your digital lives.

1. **Focus on the priority of each moment**. Try to evaluate if it's better to switch off your device completely in a given moment. Maybe you could gain some extra sleep rather than lie in bed checking your social media accounts. Or perhaps you could play with your children rather than become engrossed in a solitaire game online while they're busy with their own games on their own devices. Get into the habit of asking yourself: *What is more deserving of my attention?*

2. **Disconnect from your devices**. In order to connect with the people who matter in your life, invest in real, face-to-face contact whenever you get the chance. When you're with friends, try not to get distracted by checking your social media

accounts and replying to messages. Maybe you could switch off your phone or tablet while you're with them. Focus on having a quality connection with the person next to you, because a screen-to-screen connection will never be as nourishing as personal contact. It's the same difference as there is between nutritious, good-quality food and junk food.

3. **Turn off notifications from social media platforms**. This way your phone or computer won't send you continual alerts.

4. **Focus on balancing your chakras**. Doing so will protect your 'internal metronome of time' and your body clock. These are your internal tuning instruments and they'll help you to live your life according to your authentic 'ticking' rather than the digital 'racing pulse'. Healthy chakras will enable you to have a healthy relationship with the world around you and will prevent you from being easily overwhelmed by your environment.

5. **Connect to nature and the outside world**. Look at things with your own eyes rather than through the lens of your phone. Stop continually viewing your appreciation of nature as a potential Instagram shot that will attract lots of 'likes'. When you're outside, notice everything around you and not only from the perfect angle. Each moment and every beautiful place doesn't have to be documented for others to view! Learn how to enjoy and appreciate the world for your own nourishment and fulfilment, rather than because it's a photo opportunity or something you can post about online.

6. **Engage and contribute to the world around you**. Don't just leave a digital cloud behind you.

7. **Compile and follow a set of rules about your use of digital devices**. For example, never take your phone to bed; switch

off your phone when you're reading a book; and have a weekly 'digital rehab' in which you don't engage with your devices for a set number of hours, or even entire days.

8. **Keep your brain active.** Don't delegate every decision-making task to your computer.

9. **Send handwritten letters and cards.** Try communicating with friends and family in the traditional way, instead of sending emails and texts. We need to preserve this more personal means of communication. Buy some lovely stationery that you enjoy using, choose a beautiful pen, stock up on postage stamps, and revive the art of letter writing. Channel your words through your pen and paper, and enjoy the process.

10. **Stop relying on others' approval by collecting online 'likes'.** Instead, harness your confidence and sense of self-worth. Say the following affirmations every day, to strengthen your resolve and increase your self-esteem:

    ~   'I am enough.'

    ~   'Today, I refuse to be ruled by the opinions of others.'

    ~   'I live in the present and I'm confident about my future.'

    ~   'I'm responsible for my own happiness.'

11. **Combat metabolic stagnation.** Try daily dry-skin brushing and aerobic exercise. In my experience, when our metabolism is working fast we're less likely to resonate to stagnant 'sitting in front of the computer' energy.

When you start to take more control of your digital life, you'll also be taking more control of your life as a whole, and you'll be owning your energy rather than giving it away to a digital device.

Part V

....

THE
AURA'S
IMMUNE
SYSTEM

CHAPTER 10

Your Mechanisms of Resistance

O ur body's immune system has several layers of defence that protect it from biological pathogens. It has mechanisms in place that detect harmful intruders in our environment, block them from entering our body, attack them if they manage to penetrate us, flush out their toxins and develop future immunity to them. For example, our skin, mucus and white blood cells are all part of our immune defences. A cough, fever or diarrhoea are the immune system at work, trying to protect our body's environment.

Your Auric Skin

But did you know that the aura has an immune system too, and that it works on very similar principles to our biological one? It has the ability to spot and repel intruding harmful vibrations – the energy pathogens we talked about in Part 3 – that have the potential to interfere with our authentic frequency, deplete our auric energy reserves and generally sabotage our wellness.

Your personal space, which we discussed in Chapter 2, acts like a buffer between your inner energy system and the energy of your environment. It has an outer boundary, which can be described as an illuminated wrapping membrane that consists of energy. Some healers refer to this energetic membrane as the auric eggshell – because our personal space is often depicted as an egg, with our body in place of the egg yolk – but I call it the *auric skin*.

The auric skin is your detector of energy pathogens, and it will always try to alert you to their presence. If they aren't repelled it switches to its next line of defence, which is the filtering, protective system of your aura. And if that's not successful, these bad vibes go deeper into your inner auric system, causing it to block and stagnate, like a swelling or inflammation during an infection.

I want to emphasize that if your aura is balanced and your personal space, and its boundaries, are wholesome, then by default your natural protection will be very strong and successful in combating and stopping invading negative energy.

When you're tired, ill, stressed or emotionally and mentally low, your aura condenses, which leads to a significant reduction in the buffering of your personal space. So you lose your natural filters and your unique frequency becomes overexposed to all sorts of negative interferences. So when you set out to enhance your natural energy defence system, your primary focus should be on balancing and nourishing your aura.

Energy Protection and Clearing

My approach to protecting the aura from energy pathogens and their toxic vibrations has two aspects. When you understand my concept for energy protection you might realize why you have, until now, failed to block negative energy.

First, we must focus on balancing and strengthening our aura in order to restore our natural defence mechanisms. And second, we must perform proactive energy cleansing and protective actions: what I call *energy hygiene*. Simply focusing on remedial actions, without investing in prophylactics to boost your aura, will leave you unprotected. And vice versa.

Energy clearing is growing in popularity but, sadly, many people focus on it in acute cases, i.e. when they've already been infiltrated by negative energy. I'm inviting you to review your approach and to start by focusing on the importance of the prevention and early detection of these intruders.

I will shortly be introducing you to some of my favourite techniques for energy protection. Auric nourishment and clearing your energy filters should become your daily energy hygiene routine and part of your holistic grooming – in the same way that you brush your teeth or apply an SPF to your skin to protect it.

First, let's focus on how you commit to energy sharing and conduct your energy exchange with others, because a depleted aura equals a porous, undiscerning aura. Whenever you're in doubt about this, ask yourself: *Am I investing my energy wisely? Am I overspending my energy or am I wasting it?*

It's so important for you to be aware of how you use your energy, to understand how to strengthen the detection of harmful vibrations, and to know the energy 'cost 'of anything you commit to. Every engagement carries a price tag in the currency of your life force. Sometimes this gets repaid, but other times it doesn't. Of course, there are occasions when you don't have a choice about getting involved in an unbalanced, unreciprocated or potentially abusive energy connection, and that's when you need the protective techniques I'll be teaching you.

Always remember that no one has the power to influence and overpower you – unless, somewhere deep inside, you give them permission to do so. We *always* have a choice about whether or not to engage in an energy exchange. Yes, as I explained earlier, we have a built-in tendency to tune in to each other naturally and to form common waves, but that's not an excuse for allowing these waves to take over our unique frequency.

We can keep these energetic connections on the uppermost level of our auric skin. Only allow positive and uplifting vibrations to enter your personal space – otherwise, keep the energy exchange 'skin deep'. We must all strive to be in a state of assertive mastery, rather than in a submissive state of victimhood.

Your First Line of Defence

When we're surrounded by biological pathogens we might start to sneeze or our eyes will begin to water. This is our physical body's first line of defence; it's our immune system's way of preventing further infiltration by the irritants that are attacking us. When it happens we might choose to move away from these irritants or cover our nose with a handkerchief.

Energetically speaking, our intuition is our first line of defence. When we enter a place with negative energy or we establish a toxic connection, our intuition sends out a warning and sounds a protective alarm. In fact, it broadcasts all sorts of signals, to which we often don't pay any attention because we're only focusing on what our ego is telling us. The ego always creates a sense of urgency, causing us to forsake our awareness of and reflection on the present moment. We also don't trust our intuition when we lack confidence in ourselves.

It's important to be aware that our intuition is the first part of our aura's defence system to abandon us when our body is full of junk, which is why a healthy diet is so essential for harnessing our intuition. Without it, our inner voice will become muted by the layers of toxins we've accumulated.

Our intuition does not think. It *knows*, and it communicates with us through our senses. Sadly, this is also the reason it gets ignored, because it doesn't always resonate with our logic at that particular time. Only by looking back after some time has passed do we become aware of the bigger picture, and that's when we realize there was a hidden reason behind our 'gut feeling'.

So many of us are trapped in the realm of getting everything we want. This blocks our intuition, which is always the voice of our true needs. Like spoiled children, we hurry to fulfil our immediate desires, without stopping to reflect on the effect this might have on our authentic self or on our energy reserves.

According to a popular saying, 'You know the truth by the way it feels', and this is precisely what you should be doing: paying attention to your senses. Here are some of the most common ways our intuition communicates with us.

❖ Through our body or senses – this can include getting goose bumps, butterflies in our stomach, nausea, cold shivers, palpitations, feeling that we must get up and run away, daydream-like visions, and general uneasiness

❖ Through our dreams and in symbolic signs

❖ Through an almost audible inner voice that says things like: *This is madness* or *That feels right*

Once you've learned to recognize and trust your intuition you can use it as a tool for assessing your energy environment. Without it you'll continue to walk into energetically dirty places or connect with balance-sabotaging people.

SHARPEN YOUR INTUITION
. . . .

Here are some suggestions for becoming better acquainted with your intuition, and for sharpening it:

1. Practise silent meditations for 5–10 minutes daily – by sitting silently in a noise-free environment.

2. Cut junk food and artificial stimulants from your diet.

3. Practise alternate-nostril breathing to connect to the Sushumna meridian of now.

4. Pay attention to your third eye chakra, which governs your sixth sense and allows you to see clearly.

. . . .

Your Second Line of Defence

Your personal space is your outer 'cocoon', acting like an intermediary between your core auric energy and your environment. You might recall that I likened it to a buffer and a filter that sieves through external vibrations to protect your unique energy ID.

Your personal space is your second line of defence. You must take good care of it so it can be your haven and sanctuary. It also allows you to self-regulate whenever you're thrown off-kilter, by helping you to find and connect with your tribe of kindred spirits.

Your personal space thrives when you surround yourself with people who are on the same wavelength as you. This positive synchronization acts as a powerful natural equalizer whenever you're navigating through the toxic vibrations of problems or difficult circumstances. It will also make you a lot less inclined to form and attract toxic relationships with others.

You can probably remember a time when you were upset about something, or allowed a problem to overwhelm you, and then felt so much better after spending time with good friends, cherished family members or like-minded people. This sense of belonging is an intrinsic human need that began from a skin-to-skin contact and positive attachment with your mother or primary caregiver.

Forming positive bonds with people and other living beings – such as pets – restores our sense of perception. Balanced perception is an important tool in maintaining healthy, energetic filters. The problems and difficulties that have been looming so large and threateningly in our thoughts shrink to their proper perspective, and we may even suddenly come up with solutions to situations that had seemed all but impossible before. This protects us from accumulating the cluttered energy of unresolved problems.

Combating the State of Disconnection

Sadly, I've noticed that many of us in the Western world are increasingly suffering from a lack of auric energy protection and auric immunity as a result of a malnourished aura. This is down to the fact that we don't allocate enough importance to, nor dedicate sufficient time to, cultivating positive and genuine resonances with other people. So many people simply collect others around them, rather than *connecting* with them.

This actually weakens and clutters the aura rather than nourishing it. For example, someone might have lots of acquaintances but no one they can call a real friend. They might have hundreds of 'friends' on social media, but no one they can call if they have a problem they need to talk about or if they just want to enjoy some company.

As you probably know yourself, we can be with other people but still be lonely. It's the quality of the connection with someone that's important, not the quantity of those connections. Our phones, tablets and computers can be marvellous tools but they are increasingly isolating many of us from the rest of the world.

When you're next out and about, take a good look around you. How many people do you see who aren't looking where they're going as they walk down the street, or at those they're passing? Instead, they're gazing down at a screen, completely absorbed in what they see there, and are expecting everyone to get out of their way.

The next time you're in a bar, coffee shop or restaurant, notice how many people are physically together but emotionally disconnected. They aren't talking to one another; instead, each is lost in their own little world as they stare at the screen on their phone or tablet. And it's the same in many people's homes, with everyone glued to their particular device and no one speaking. In some households, people will even text each other to ask questions or make comments instead of having a face-to-face conversation!

This sort of emotional disconnection might seem like an increasingly normal part of life but it leads to a chronic deficiency in our aura. Loneliness has now reached epidemic proportions in many countries, with millions identifying themselves as lonely and starved of genuine and high-quality contact with other humans.

See if you can devote more time to face-to-face conversations, rather than screen-to-screen chats. Even simple actions, which might not seem very important at all, can have a big impact on us. For instance, making eye contact with the person who serves you in a shop and smiling at them can transform what might otherwise be an anonymous experience into something sincere and personal.

Pay attention to the people you attract into your life and make an effort to get to know them. Try not to focus on clichéd questions about where they're from or what they do for a living, and instead ask about their passions and experiences.

It's always enriching to form a positive bond with people by engaging in activities that serve others or a higher good in the world, such as volunteering. Shared goals and values create positive waves that boost your energy space.

Please note that solitude and loneliness are not the same. Solitude, when self-imposed and temporary, is a state of connection – connection to the soul – and it can be a very enriching and fortifying experience. Loneliness is quite the opposite, as it's a state of disconnection and deficiency.

Gatekeepers of Your Truth

As I mentioned earlier, our personal space is defined by its outer boundary, or auric skin, which also makes up part of our second line of defence. Once again, when your aura is well balanced and resonating with your authentic frequency, this outer membrane has an elastic quality that repels dissonant vibrations.

However, I would like to mention here that healthy psychological boundaries are an essential part of your aura's immune system. With your intuition as the first line of defence, you'll have an awareness of what resonates with your authentic frequency and what doesn't.

Based on this, you can learn to speak your truth by verbally drawing lines with the words 'yes' or 'no'. Just as loneliness compromises our personal space, saying 'yes' to something when we mean to say 'no' rips our auric skin apart and exposes our aura to abuse. Don't look at your boundaries as a structure that blocks other people. A healthier perspective is to view them as a mechanism to stop *you* from compromising yourself and from ending up in an energetically toxic environment. Look at your boundaries as the gatekeepers of your truth and of your authentic life force.

Now that you're familiar with the principles of your aura's immune system, we can go deeper and start looking into the subject of protection in greater detail. I shall share with you my favourite tips for taking care of your layers of defence.

Above all, I'll show you how to boost your aura and attune it to its unique frequency, so you can only attract what's truly yours. This is absolutely essential for owning your energy because if you're not protected you're owned by the traffic of intruding waves and will lose your energy ID. And, as you're now aware, this will put an end to any attempts at achieving sustainable wellness.

So, let's get practical!

CHAPTER 11

Strategies for Effective Protection

In the remainder of this part of the book I'll be teaching you useful exercises for protecting yourself from toxic energy. But first I'd like to give you some tips on how to do them properly. Like so many things in life, mastering the correct application of a technique makes a huge difference to the end result.

How to Visualize and Meditate Correctly

Often, we don't train ourselves to perform guided visualizations and meditations in the right way, and tend to use surrogate versions that have limited benefits. Refining your ability to visualize and meditate can reap many rewards.

Step 1: 'Touch' an Object with Your Vision

First of all, you need to practise expanding your *imagination*, which is one of the most powerful tools in energy work, meditation and visualization. You're going to touch an object, first with your fingers and then only with your vision. You can choose any object, such as a table or a vase of flowers, but it's best to focus on an inanimate one rather than a pet, which may move and distract you.

Intention: to train your imagination. If you don't master this technique you won't be able to follow guided visualizations effectively. Instead, you'll do them in a one-dimensional way, and they won't work properly.

It's very important to keep your eyes open during this technique. Do it for one or two minutes at a time, two or three times a day, for one week, and each time focus on a different object.

1. Start by choosing the object you want to concentrate on.

2. Handle it, so you know how it feels in as many ways as possible.

3. Now sit with the object near you, and 'touch' it with your eyes. Let your imagination tell you how it feels. Sense its weight, whether it's warm or cold, how its surface feels. Is it shiny or matt? Does it have a pleasing texture? Imagine everything about it in as much detail as possible.

4. After one or two minutes, mentally put the object back where you found it.

Step 2: Create Your Energy Twin

Next, you're going to visually create your *energy twin* as your inner helper. This is a miniature version of yourself, and you'll be using it here and in another exercise later. If you wish, you can give it a different name than energy twin: just make sure it's a positive one with positive connotations for you. It's your miniature, imagined double, which you'll accept as your energy 'mini-me'. You can also visualize and refer to it by name instead of visualizing deities any time you pray for strength or help. It will cultivate your trust in your unlimited inner resources and harness the belief that you are enough.

Intention: to visually create a vivid energy form of your miniature 'double'.

1. Sit quietly and close your eyes.

2. Mentally hold out the palm of your dominant hand (if it helps, you can hold out your actual palm) and imagine a miniature version of yourself sitting on it.

3. Visualize yourself in as much vivid and positive detail as possible, including your hair, face and body. Imagine that your energy twin is wearing some of your favourite clothes and is smiling at you. Smile back!

4. Mentally thank your energy twin for 'materializing' and ask them to reappear whenever you call on their help.

5. Imagine your energy twin dematerializing, and then slowly open your eyes.

Step 3: Create An Intention

Many people forget this step, yet it's essential. Intention creates the vessel for receiving, and it means you always predetermine what you attract. So make sure that you always create the intention for your meditation or guided visualization.

State your intention clearly in your mind before proceeding with any form of energy practice. For instance, you might want to do a guided visualization with the intention of feeling relaxed or being protected. So, say in your head: *I dedicate this meditation to my relaxation* or *I intend to protect my aura with this visualization.*

Step 4: Say Affirmations Correctly

Here's another very important step that not everyone knows about: always say your affirmations in your mother tongue: the language you used during the formative years (the first eight to ten) of your life. Your aura and subconscious mind will generate much stronger feedback to this.

Affirmations are even more powerful when you say them out loud while looking at your reflection in a mirror. I'd also recommend you use your non-dominant hand when writing your affirmations on a piece of paper. It might not look as pretty but it'll be more effective.

Be very careful about the words you use for your affirmations. Make sure that they're always positive and don't carry any sort of negative charge. For instance, if you want to recover from an illness, you mustn't refer to that illness in your affirmation. This is because your subconscious will register the illness and want to give you more of it, which of course is the last thing you want. Always choose a positive way of affirming what you want, based on your ultimate objective rather than a problem that you're trying to overcome. Here are some examples of positive affirmations:

❖ 'I'm full of energy' instead of 'I'm not tired'.

❖ 'I have abundance' instead of 'I need more money'.

❖ 'I'm completely healthy' instead of 'I'm not ill'.

❖ 'My life is full of joy' instead of 'I'm not sad'.

How to End Meditations

Meditation and visualization exercises become more powerful if you combine them with physical activity. This is because you're engaging both the left and right hemispheres of the brain; and besides, Westerners find it easier to meditate when they combine it with action. You'll find that many of the exercises in this book incorporate both physical and imagined activities. My special way of ending meditations also combines these elements:

❖ Towards the end of a meditation, stand up and, keeping your eyes closed and your feet static, sway your body as though it's a pendulum for around 15–20 seconds.

❖ While you do this, imagine that you're inside a swirling, rainbow-coloured spiral of energy, like a whirligig toy.

❖ Now say, 'I am in the energy flow. I am protected by the energy flow. I am the flow.' Then open your eyes.

This is a very good way to anchor yourself in lightness and protection, regardless of the intention behind your practice. If you prefer, you can end your meditations while sitting down and swaying your upper body. You can do this in bed too, if you wish. Simply do as much as your physical ability allows.

The Power of Disengagement

As we've discussed, tuning in to others is a natural, healthy and instinctive ability for us. But this doesn't mean we have to become a victim, ruled by other people's energies and demands 24 hours a day. Like any other of our special senses, this ability has to serve us. This means we should cultivate our sensitivity to energy but not approach it with fear or any other overreaction.

It's a question of vibrational *observation* versus vibrational *engagement*. Observing something, so that you have some distance from it and exercise your discernment, is different from being automatically engaged with it. I often find that my patients are scared of the increased sensitivity or enhanced intuition that comes from their healing sessions, yet these are their best allies in employing authentic forces for their protection. Just as we don't make ourselves blind when we see something unpleasant, so we shouldn't make ourselves vibrationally numb to anything difficult that we experience in our lives.

As I've already explained, we have choice and awareness. This means we have the choice to leave a situation or a person when we're unhappy, so we don't have to experience it or them any longer. Sometimes, of course, we can't leave, which is when we can create a 'neutral state' (I'll be showing you how to do that shortly). Once again, remember that nothing can affect you unless you give it permission to do so. Being surrounded by toxic energy doesn't mean it has to penetrate and become part of you. In any circumstances you have the power to remain strong, rooted and whole.

Observer Meditations

Here are two meditations that will help you to observe your life without being distracted or influenced by your reactions or emotions. Before you perform either of them, you need the intention to understand *why* you're doing them. So the correct preparation for each meditation is as important as the meditation itself.

Both meditations require you to use your imagination, and you may struggle with this at first if you're unfamiliar with using your imagination fully. Use the step-by-step exercise at the start of this chapter to help you develop your imagination. Keep at it, because it takes time to build up your imagination muscle.

Don't despair and don't be hard on yourself. Start with images that work for you and trust that your intention to perform these meditations will be beneficial for you – even if, at first, you feel you aren't doing them as well as you'd like. The more senses you involve in your visualizations, the more potent they will become.

We need to cultivate the state of an observer because it may not come naturally any longer, especially when we're exposed to lots of outer stimuli that we can't control. Think of the observer state as like a default setting on your personal computer. Whenever you feel overwhelmed, you can restore your default setting to neutral. This is one of the best ways to take care of your personal space, which is at its most powerful and protective when you're in the state of an observer.

THE NEUTRAL STATE

You can sit or stand for this meditation. Set aside a time when you won't be disturbed or distracted, so you can completely immerse yourself in it. Keep practising it until you can enter the neutral state at will.

Intention: to create a sense of harmony, and to foster a neutral state that allows you to protect yourself, boost your energy, and deflect any emotional pressures that others may try to place on you.

✧ Imagine your energy twin (see step 2 at the beginning of the chapter).

✧ Now imagine it standing on top of your head. Make sure your energy twin is small enough that it can easily descend into and through your bigger (physical) self. Shift your consciousness and awareness into your energy twin. Identify with it fully.

✧ Slowly and gradually, you find yourself descending on a parachute into your larger self's head. Once inside, you find yourself floating down through the clouds. They can be foggy or cloudy. You may see lots of lightning and hear thunder. Now imagine rays of sunlight coming through the dark clouds as you move slowly, so slowly, down.

✧ You reach the level of your larger self's throat, your neck, and now you're floating through blue sky, gliding lower and lower – slowly through your throat area and down through your shoulders and chest. At the level of your stomach, you land on the ground, feeling its softness and warmth. The freshness of the green aromatic herbs there relaxes you. Then you continue downwards.

✧ Just below the level of your navel, you find a beautiful, quiet lake with a little boat waiting at its edge. You get into the boat and sit down, and it then sails off onto the still waters.

✧ From your boat you look down into the water and at the water lilies floating there. Have you ever seen water lilies, the way they float, their petals opening? It's impossible to compare this view with anything else. It deserves your undivided attention a little longer, so just observe: don't think about anything else. Stay inside your internal world. Rest inside the world of yourself. Observe your breath.

✧ You're breathing almost through the top of your head. Through the top of your head, you inhale air from the surrounding environment; the air of higher levels, free from the energy of other people. It's almost as if you have a hollow pillar on top of your head, which is light in both colour and weight. It allows you to pull down the air from the higher levels of the atmosphere.

✧   Together with the air, you absorb light and then inhale the light inside yourself. Allow the little self that's resting so beautifully inside you, on that blue lake of your inner world, to take the beautiful light as a precious gift.

. . . .

The following exercise is another very good one for creating a neutral state, especially when you're presented with challenging situations.

THE PERISCOPE

After you've practised this and the previous exercise, you can decide which one you prefer. You might want to mix and match, depending on your circumstances.

Intention: to enable you to look at the bigger picture of any situation, so you can deal with it wisely and with a sense of detachment.

1.   Imagine that you're pulling a periscope out of the crown chakra on the top of your head. Keep pulling it until it's about 1 m (3 ft) tall.

2.   Next, look at your external world through the top of the periscope. Note how different everything looks from this very different perspective.

3. Now, every time you're presented with a difficult situation, immediately pull out your 'periscope' and use it to observe what's going on. You'll find you're able to resolve the situation much more easily, and in a wise and detached manner.

From time to time pull out your 'periscope' and view your life through its thin glass, as if you're viewing a movie from an auditorium. This will give you a much better and less cluttered view of your problems and circumstances.

. . . .

Changing Your Attitude

When we have choice and awareness, we can often free and unburden ourselves by changing our attitude to an event or a person that has been causing us grief, regret or anger. Many of the things that happen to us in life are actually neutral – the events themselves are neither positive nor negative, it's our *attitude* towards them that makes them seem good or bad. Of course, there are times when we are faced with real tragedy.

We can attach many different emotions to a person or an event but often we project a negative attitude towards them because we're feeling annoyed or tired, or because they remind us of something difficult that happened in the past. This is often an instinctive reaction but it doesn't have to be an automatic response. Our attitude towards people and circumstances doesn't happen without us making a *choice* about how we view them or present them to ourselves.

Try to train yourself to have a neutral 'pause' before forming an attitude. Or you might adapt the life approach of one of my friends, who says: 'I tend to view everything positively unless proven otherwise.'

See the Bigger Picture

My favourite of the Dalai Lama's sayings is: 'Sometimes not getting what you want is a wonderful stroke of luck'. At times, especially when we feel disappointed or dejected about things not working out in the way we wanted, the bigger picture eludes us.

It's only later in life that we're given an insight into why something played out the way it did, and that it was ultimately for our benefit – even if we weren't aware of it at the time. We always have to allow for a different possibility from the one we've planned or were hoping for; and we need to realize that our perception can be blinkered because the Universe is not yet showing us the full picture. We may only see a fraction of it.

Sometimes, while you're focusing on what you want, your auric skin is repelling something that could be potentially very damaging to your *true* needs. In any case, as we Russians say, 'Everything that happens, happens for the best!'

Rehashing the Past

Do you often go over past events in your mind? Do you tend to dwell on the difficult things that have happened to you, rather than the good ones? It's so important not to let past hurts cross the boundaries of what's happening right now. These experiences may have hurt you badly but they are ghosts of the past and aren't happening to you any longer.

Often, a tendency to dwell on the event is much more damaging than the event itself. Resentment can eat into your soul because you're the one whose energy is being affected by it, not the person or event you resent. As Nelson Mandela said, 'Resentment is like drinking poison and then hoping it will kill your enemies.'

Yogic alternate-nostril breathing is very beneficial in this case as it shifts you from the dominance of the Ida meridian of the past into the Sushumna meridian of now. You can also try the following meditation.

SHINE A LIGHT

This is a good meditation for switching off mentally and emotionally from any traumatic or difficult situation that you keep thinking about. Choose a time when you can be alone and won't be disturbed. Turn off all electronic devices so they won't interrupt or distract you.

Intention: to help you heal your emotional response to a situation that occurred in your past.

✧ Sit comfortably in a chair or in your favourite meditation pose. Take three deep breaths and feel yourself relaxing. Close your eyes.

✧ Imagine that you're in a theatre and the traumatic or upsetting event is playing out on a stage in front of you while you watch it from the dark auditorium.

✧ Imagine that you see all the people involved in the past event, including yourself, but still retain your view as the observer, sitting in the auditorium.

✧ Now imagine that the 'observer you' in the auditorium is holding a torch. Hold it up, switch it on and direct it at the action unfolding on stage. The torch is shining on what's happening with a light so bright that it's almost dazzling. Spend time surrounding the scene with this light until you no longer feel emotionally consumed by the event and naturally shift into a state of neutral disengaged observation.

✧ When you're ready, switch off the torch and walk out of the auditorium.

✧ Come back into your body and be present in the room once again.

. . . .

After practising this exercise you'll still be able to remember the difficult situation but you'll have removed its emotional 'colouring', and that's what's important. The situation will start to loosen its energetic grip on you.

CHAPTER 12

Safeguarding Barriers

Before you begin a messy or dirty task, do you put on protective gloves or clothes? Maybe you wear rubber gloves when doing the washing-up or housework, put on an apron before you start cooking or a breathing mask when you're tackling a job that creates clouds of dust?

These all are barriers that provide physical protection, preventing us from getting dirty and keeping germs from penetrating deep into our body. You now know that our aura also requires protective barriers when it's exposed to energy pathogens. These also act as prophylactics against wider contamination.

I want you to become the master of each moment, and that means owning your energy and getting out your protective shield if something is threatening the authentic flow of your energy. You must also be able to shake off or neutralize any harmful vibrations that become attached to your auric skin, so this 'splinter' of negative energy doesn't travel further into your aura.

I've noticed that people often approach the subject of energy protection with fear and submissive vulnerability. It's worth remembering that the emotion of fear trips us into a knocked-out state – like a boxer who has adopted a defeatist position even before the match begins. So I'd like to encourage you to apply energy protection techniques with no more emotion than you have when pulling on rubber gloves or taking a shower. Just view the tips in this chapter as a part of your general hygiene habits – which, as you've learned, must be broadened to allow for energy protection and clearing.

Wield Your Shield

Here are two 'shielding' techniques you can use during the types of attack on your aura that happen most frequently.

LACE OF LIGHT

This is a lovely protective exercise that my mother taught me. When you first use it, allow plenty of time, so you can do it fully. With more practice you'll be able to manifest this protection almost instantly.

Intention: to protect your authentic vibrations in a beautiful way, especially before you enter a difficult environment.

1. Close your eyes. Imagine a small golden sphere hovering above the crown of your head. Imagine the sphere slowly starting to spin in a clockwise direction, making a very small circle. As it moves it leaves traces of iridescent light behind it, like a sparkler.

2. Now imagine the golden sphere moving in all sorts of directions as it weaves around your head. Soon those

shimmering traces of light it leaves in its wake form an intricate, lace-like pattern around your aura.

3. Continue to imagine the golden sphere as it moves down around your body, weaving an ornate network of fine, delicate, light-filled lace around your aura. Don't forget the areas of your body that you can't see, such as the back of your head and neck, your back, the backs of your legs and the soles of your feet.

4. Allow the protective network of glowing lace to cover your entire aura, like a beautifully wrapped auric cocoon, and then seal it by imagining that you're signing your name in light on it. Just write your name, like an artist marking his masterpiece.

5. When you're about to enter an environment that you find threatening or really challenging, make your lace of light tighter, with fewer holes.

. . . .

The next exercise is a superfast and simple way of sealing your aura.

DIAMOND PROTECTION

The Diamond Protection doesn't require visualization so you can practise it in any situation, even during meetings or conversations. What's more, you can do it discreetly, so no one notices what you're doing.

Intention: this exercise closes your auric circuit so no energy can leak and drain out of you. This makes you less susceptible to other people's neediness or attacks, and you become energetically unavailable for any kind of parasitic attachment.

1. Sit, and rest your hands comfortably on your thighs.

2. Place the tip of your tongue behind your top teeth, at the point where they meet the roof of your mouth.

3. Place the tips of your thumbs together so they point up towards your solar plexus, and at the same time, place the tips of your two index fingers together so they are pointing in front of you. Your thumbs and index fingers should form a teardrop shape.

4. Allow your remaining fingers to curl around each other, with those of the right hand on top of the left. This protective 'diamond' hand gesture, combined with the tongue–front teeth connection, will put your aura on instant lockdown.

. . . .

Strategies for Acute Protection

Here are some very effective strategies and exercises to help you protect your aura from your opponent's 'thorns' and their damage during a negative energy exchange.

Protect your Solar Plexus

You might recall that your solar plexus chakra governs your social interactions. So, the first punch from a negative energy exchange with another person often lands on this energy centre. If someone starts to attack or criticize you, especially out of the blue, take immediate avoiding action by placing something over your solar plexus. This creates a physical barrier between you and the person attacking you.

Of course, you must do this in a way that seems perfectly natural, rather than defensive. If you're sitting down, get to your feet and stand behind a chair or sofa, or a similar object nearby. Sometimes that isn't possible, so reach out for a cushion to hug instead, or even a jacket that you can hold against your tummy. It will look like a completely natural and spontaneous action, but you'll know that your intention is to protect your solar plexus from energetic attack.

If you wear an amulet or crystals for protection they should be on a chain long enough that the pendant rests on your solar plexus chakra. Very often, people don't achieve the full benefits from these spiritual tools for protection because they place them on the chest, which is a lot higher than the solar plexus.

Do Something Unexpected

Another important protective action during a verbal attack is to do something that the other person isn't expecting, so you break the template of behaviour that they expect from you. You could bend down and rearrange your shoelaces, pull up your socks, shuffle pieces of paper around on your desk, start watering the houseplants, or anything else that seems appropriate but doesn't relate to your opponent's behaviour or expectations, or what they're talking about.

Don't do this nervously, anxiously or angrily – try to be as natural as possible. Your opponent will be expecting you to shout back or respond with some other form of aggression or submissiveness; in other words they will want to get a 'fix' from your reaction. When you do something totally different, they'll be thrown off-kilter. Don't worry if they're confused by what you're doing because, from your point of view, that's a good thing. When we're confused our energy field becomes weak and disjointed, which often leads to a much less forceful and less confident impact on others.

Slow Down

If someone is verbally attacking you, minimize the auric damage this will cause by slowing down the up-flow of your inner energy. To do this, hold your breath or significantly slow down your breathing while the insults are being thrown at you. This will act as metaphorical earplugs for your aura.

Stay Calm

Don't respond to provocation from another person. If you do, you'll be trapped in an endless cycle of absorbing their negativity or releasing your emotional energy for their gratification. When this happens, people will keep baiting and feeding from you. If you stay calm and don't respond to their provocations, you'll be in control of the energy exchange. Own your energy and control your emotional responses, even when you're manipulated to get a reaction while your buttons are being pressed.

Don't shrivel up just because someone decides to belittle or humiliate you; don't take offence when someone tries to offend you; and don't get angry when someone goads you. The bottom line is simple – don't respond to every emotional stimulation or provocation. Don't allow negative people to turn you into one of them.

Change the Tone

If someone is shouting at you or verbally attacking you, calmly and confidently ask them to take a step back. Most of the time, that person will do as you ask, which in turn will make you less submissive to their negative influence and enable you to gain control over the energy exchange and reinforce your personal space.

Alternatively, don't respond to or comment on what the person is saying, and ask them to alter their tone instead. In this way you treat the essence of their words with indifference and only ask them to adjust the frequency of their voice. For example, you could ask, 'Please can you tell me what you'd like to say in a calmer or quieter voice?'

Keep It Formal

If you have a tendency to become involved in negative energy exchanges with a certain person or sense passive aggression from them – especially if you encounter them through your work – if possible, try to avoid being on first-name terms with them. Address them, and ask to be addressed as, Mr, Mrs or Ms so-and-so, or whatever is appropriate.

Try an Inner Smile

If someone is being very intimidating or passively aggressive, and you feel oppressed by their negative presence, imagine that they're smiling at you, *or* imagine them as a baby. This will uplift the energy flow between you and prevent any feelings of submissive vulnerability. Alternatively, you can relax and smile an inner smile: one that isn't obvious but which you know is radiating within you. In your mind, wish that person happiness, and then exhale with a sigh. You will then remain the master of your energy space.

Avoid Someone's Gaze

There's a saying in Russia and also in Britain that the eyes are the windows of the soul. That's why you should never look someone in the eye if they're attacking you verbally or energetically. Instead, keep your gaze just above the bridge of their nose (which is the location of the third eye chakra), otherwise your core energy will be a lot more exposed and vulnerable to the negative vibrations of their outburst.

Auric Holes

During a heated argument or an aggressive verbal exchange with someone, both your and their aura swells and expands. Each aura starts to spin very fast and in a chaotic and turbulent way. Its usually soft, glowing rays turn into thorn-like spikes of energy that inflict emotional and spiritual wounds on both you and your opponent.

This kind of auric distortion also happens one-sidedly to the aura of the person who is angrily aggravated and launching a verbal and emotional attack on you and, as a result, perforates your aura. Energy vampires also tend to damage your aura by piercing it like a mosquito or, in some cases, slicing it with the vibrations of their sharp words. That's why we explored the subject of energy vampires in such detail earlier, because your first step towards protecting yourself against them is recognizing them in your environment.

If we don't mend these auric 'holes' that develop from difficult connections with others, our energy will continue to leach out of them; and, no matter how often we replenish our reserves, it will soon drain away again – making this another sabotaging factor in our bid for sustainable wellness.

Sadly, so many people are walking around with their aura 'bleeding' energy through multiple ruptures. This happens because they aren't aware of the aura damage that happens during a negative energy exchange and therefore are not protecting or repairing their energy field.

All these energy leaks continue unnoticed for a very long time, until they accumulate and leave us absolutely drained and depressed. We simply lose any ability to retain our energy, regardless of how many times we try to replenish it. It's like a boat developing a hole in its hull – water will slowly seep into the boat until it eventually sinks. That's what happens with small problems and setbacks: each one may seem minor, but collectively they can sink us.

Spotting Auric Holes

These are the most common manifestations of energy holes in your aura:

❖ **Extreme empathy**: you feel like a sponge, picking up all the energy around you. Your sensitivity overwhelms and totally governs your internal state. You feel touched by everything you hear from people or the media.

❖ **Feeling unsafe**: being on your own makes you feel vulnerable, while at the same time, being with a crowd makes you feel exposed. You just want to stay indoors, yet you surround yourself with friends and family. It's almost as though you're using their energy to fill your inner void. It's your subconscious desire to plug that auric hole.

❖ **Lack of stamina**: the loss of your normal zest and vitality. You might feel uncharacteristically flat, emotionally, or depressed.

Tending to Your Auric Wounds

Now that you have a better awareness of the implications for your aura of a negative interpersonal exchange we can look at tending to your auric 'wounds' so they stop becoming an entry point for energy pathogens and an exit for your life force. It's worth mentioning, too, that these auric holes also appear when we produce toxic vibrations from synchronizing with destructive waves, as we discussed earlier in the book.

Identify Your Ruptured Chakra

We'll use the chakra system to repair a newly formed hole after an attack. So, pick the chakra that's the most appropriate to your current situation from the following list. I've also included here a reminder of the colours that I associate with each of the chakras; you'll need to refer to these when you practise the *Mend Your Aura* exercise opposite.

Base Chakra: conflict based on domestic or family-related problems; pressure for impulsive actions, not those that are thought through; threats to your safety: and exchange with a Paranoid vampire. *Colour:* ruby red.

Navel Chakra: an attack on your sexuality, woman-/manhood; rape; an outburst of jealousy or envy directed at you; the accusation that you don't deserve something; an exchange with a Green-Eyed Monster vampire. *Colour:* orange-gold.

Solar Plexus Chakra: the projection of someone else's responsibility onto you; pressure to abandon your path and follow someone else's; an emotionally threatening environment; your opponent's anger because you don't live up to their expectations; an exchange with an Emotional Blackmailer or Temporary vampire. *Colour:* yellow-gold.

Heart Chakra: betrayal of your love; a verbal outburst directed at you which states that you're not worthy of love; frequent close contact with a Peacock or Smother Love vampire. *Colour:* grass green.

Throat Chakra: when someone metaphorically pushes their words down your throat; projections of guilt; denial by others of your right to speak; the company of a Full-On Chatterbox vampire. *Colour:* turquoise.

Third Eye Chakra: verbal assaults on your wisdom and insights; passive-aggressive behaviour that belittles and ridicules your intuition; an attack by a Bully vampire. *Colour:* Indigo blue.

Crown Chakra: outbursts that accuse you of being stupid; an attack on your identity; an argument about your spiritual practices; an exchange with a Manipulator vampire. *Colour:* white, violet.

MEND YOUR AURA

As I've already mentioned, visualizations are most potent when combined with physical movement, so for this energy exercise, you can use your hands to make small 'sewing' actions. If that isn't possible you can use this simply as a visualization.

You can either sit or stand for this exercise, depending on the position of the auric hole that you want to mend. See Chapter 1 for the locations of the chakras and their characteristics.

Intention: applying first aid to the damage from a negative energy exchange; use it to 'sew up' the holes in your aura so your energy no longer leaks out of them.

✧ Close your eyes, bring your awareness to the relevant chakra and imagine what the hole in it looks like. Is it a small rip, a larger tear or a gaping hole?

✧ Imagine that you're holding a golden needle between your index finger and your thumb. Picture an array of cotton reels and choose the colour of the thread that matches the colour of the chakra associated with the symptoms you're experiencing. Thread the golden needle with your chosen cotton.

✧ Now imagine that you're carefully darning the hole in your aura. Use neat, small stitches and keep sewing until the hole is completely closed. Really visualize the way the opening becomes smaller and smaller with each movement of the needle.

✧ When you've finished sewing up the hole, in your mind's eye vividly see that it's completely and tightly closed. Stroke that area of your aura with your hand (you can actually put your hand on your body where the chakra is located) and imagine that you're ironing it flat using your palm's golden light until all the stitches have disappeared and you only see the smooth, homogenous glow of the chakra's colour.

. . . .

Family Energy Protection

If you encounter a lot of difficult people in your workplace or in a social setting, you may be able to avoid them or find other strategies for keeping them at arm's length. But what do you do if your partner or a member of the family needles you and feeds off your energy?

Often, energy loss in a family happens during conflicts and arguments. There may be lots of verbal exchanges and emotional flare-ups, and they can be incredibly energy sapping if we don't know how to deal with them or realize that we can choose how to respond.

Now is Not the Time...

We all need to remember to respond to others' states and provocations wisely. For instance, if your partner comes home in a bad mood and they're obviously on edge, you need to tune in to this and realize that it probably isn't the best moment to say something that will trigger a row, such as showing them the latest domestic bill or announcing that their least favourite guest is coming to stay for the weekend.

If they are really irritable and not ready to talk to you about anything, it might even be best to leave them alone and go into another room, or head off for a walk. Otherwise, they'll have a strong reaction to whatever you say, which will damage you and inevitably lead to energy loss.

Drop Your Voice

Once again, pay attention to the tone of your voice. When someone you live with starts shouting at you, don't shout back.

Their energy loss is their choice. Keep your own energy loss to a minimum by lowering your voice and speaking quietly. Make sure you don't speak at the same tempo as the other person or you'll form a toxic common wavelength. If you can drop your voice by a couple of octaves, it will keep you composed and invincible.

Dealing With a Victim

What should you do when a partner or family member comes home, having had an awful day, and keeps on venting and complaining, as though they're a victim of what happened? Often we sit and listen, soaking up their irritation and distress like sponges. Although this might seem supportive, it feeds the person's tendency to dwell on how things have gone wrong for them.

I don't advocate doing this. I think you should show empathy towards them and validate their feelings, but then turn the conversation round so it's more proactive than stagnant. For instance, you could say 'I hear you. I'm sorry about what's happened. Let's see how it can be resolved. How are you planning to deal with the situation?'

Making positive suggestions about how to improve the situation and asking about their action plan, instead of reinforcing their sense of victimhood, helps them to kick-start their third eye chakra, which is the one that's responsible for creating tactics and strategies and being proactive. I always advise my patients to do this if they don't want to be an energetic rubbish bin for someone else's negative energy or feelings.

Being a container for someone's bad energy doesn't help them and it certainly doesn't help you! You don't need to prove your love and friendship by drowning yourself when you're with someone who's already drowning. Instead, help them up by focusing on the forward-moving energy of the future. Remember, there's a huge difference between helping someone and sacrificing yourself for them.

Ending an Argument

We all need to remember the saying 'Never go to bed on an argument'. It's so important, especially with family members, to talk things through and release them before you go to bed. Then you can allow your energy to repair itself overnight. If you don't do this, you won't have a restful night's sleep because you'll still be holding on to all that negative energy.

If you have a major argument with your partner and you both feel real animosity towards each other, with no prospect of making up your differences immediately, try to sleep in separate rooms that night. If you share a bed when you feel furious with one another, you'll damage each other's aura even more than you already have and will literally sleep on a bed of energetic thorns.

Sometimes it's impossible to sleep separately, in which case, when in bed you should imagine that you've drawn an invisible curtain between the two of you. Remember to remove it in the morning because I want you to start your new day with the chance of a reconnection.

More Tools for Aura Protection

Here are some more beautifully simple but highly effective visualizations, meditations and other exercises for protecting your aura.

RIBBON PROTECTION

Intention: to seal your aura and protect yourself when dealing with energy pathogens.

When in the presence of an energy vampire or simply a negative person, mentally place yourself inside a sphere that's filled with beautiful amethyst-hued light. The outside of this sphere is wrapped in rainbow-coloured ribbons, just like an exquisite gift. Imagine that each ribbon has writing on it saying, 'I am protected', 'I am invincible', 'I am safe'.

Using the ribbon protection visualization will make it a lot harder for the intruding energy to violate your personal space.

BRICK WALL PROTECTION

Intention: to block negative energy from entering your personal space.

If you're with someone who bullies, provokes or energetically attacks you, imagine a brick wall being built between the two of you. The side of the wall facing the other person is covered with a mirror, so they can only see their own reflection. Any negative energy projected by that person will therefore be reflected back to them, instead of reaching you.

When you're no longer with this person, or if you no longer feel they're attacking you, don't stay in an energetically defensive state.

. . . .

When exposed to negative and hostile energy, the following exercise will prevent you from being saturated in toxic waves.

BECOME TRANSPARENT
. . . .

Intention: to prevent negative energy latching onto you.

✧ First, induce the neutral state of the observer, which I described in Chapter 11.

✧ Then imagine that you're completely transparent and the currents of negative energy are flowing through you without stopping and without you catching them. In your head, say, *I am invisible to toxic energy*.

✧ You can then imagine that all the negative energy, which has passed through you, turns into a pink mist. Either picture it dissipating or being absorbed into the ground – whichever image works best for you. This will be a lovely act of space-clearing, even if it was someone else who energetically littered and not you.

. . . .

Do the following Burning Matches exercise when you've been a victim of a negative exchange – I guess we all know how heavy we feel afterwards, but it's amazing how much this technique can help.

BURNING MATCHES

Before you begin, you'll need to buy some extra-long matches – the sort that are made for lighting barbecues and open fires (a lighter isn't suitable).

Intention: to clear yourself quickly of negative energy caused by a difficult situation or emotion.

1.   Strike a match. While looking at the flame create the intention to release yourself from the burden of an emotion and a situation that still grips you.

2.   Hold on to the intention, then exhale and blow out the match with a sigh – an 'ahh', rather than a puff.

3.   Now throw away the match.

Energy Clearing

Sometimes we fail to protect ourselves from the negative energy of people or events, and end up feeling as though we've been infected by it. In Russia we say that 'habit becomes a character' and in my practice I often see old toxic energy build-up become accepted as a part of the Self. So, it's important to clear it as soon as you detect its accumulation. You can use the visualizations that follow to self-regulate with energy clearing.

COMBING THE AURA

This is a really effective exercise for clearing your aura of all the negative energy it's picked up. You can do it whenever you need to, but especially if you've just had an unpleasant experience or have been talking to a difficult person and feel as though you can't remove 'the dirty footsteps' of their energy from your aura.

This combines physical movements and visualization, for maximum effectiveness. The more tuned in you are to energy, the more you'll sense the benefits of this exercise.

Intention: to clean and purify your aura by 'combing it'.

1. Imagine that you're holding a comb made from pure gold. It feels warm and is glowing in your hand.

2. Starting with the aura around your head, pull the golden comb through each section of it. Don't forget the back of your head and the crown.

3. Continue down your body, combing the aura around your neck and shoulders, along each arm to your fingertips, down your trunk, down your hips, between your legs, down each leg to your toes and to the soles of your feet.

4. While you do this, imagine a burning violet flame beside you, ready to receive the negative energy you're extracting from your aura.

5. Whenever you feel that your comb is full of the dark energetic fluff you've removed from your aura, pull it out with your hands and drop it into the heart of the violet flame.

6. Keep doing this until you've combed your entire aura. Now ask the violet flame to drift away and return to the universal light source.

You can combine this visualization with an actual hand movement, using your fingers as the teeth of the visualized comb. Move your hand in a brisk combing motion, following the guidance for the visualization, and lightly touch your body as if removing the balls of fluff from yourself.

. . . .

Earlier, you learned about auric 'bacteria' or energy cords. You've probably already reflected on whether you're infected with this kind of pathogen and, if so, have established which chakra is affected; try the following exercise to burn your cord(s).

BURNING ENERGY CORDS

Intention: freeing yourself from negative attachments.

✧ Prepare a candle (a church candle or tea light) and a match and place them in front of you.

✧ Imagine the person whom you feel has formed a negative attachment with you.

✧ Now bring your awareness to the affected chakra and imagine that a coloured thread (matching the colour of the chakra; see pages 16–22) is stretching between your chakra and theirs. Stay with this feeling, making it as vivid as possible.

✧ Now open your eyes, light the candle in front of you and close your eyes once again, returning to the previous visualization.

✧ Imagine now that you're lighting the coloured thread, which acts like a sparkler. The burning sparks are travelling along the thread towards the person and leave no trace behind.

✧ Once the sparks finally reach the other end of the thread, at that person's chakra, they create a very bright explosion of light between you, after which you're both completely covered in a cloud of shining white mist.

✧ Now open your eyes, pick up the burning candle and move it in front of you at a distance of 30–50 cm (12–20 inches) from your body, starting at the base chakra and finishing at the crown chakra.

✧ Say 'I release you into the hands of light and love. I am free and restored.' Then place the candle somewhere safe and allow it to burn until it goes out.

. . . .

The following exercise is great for neutralizing energy.

WASH IT OFF!

After you arrive home, have a shower as soon as possible, so you can literally wash off the energy you've accumulated over the day. Let the water cascade over the crown of your head and down your entire body, because the negative energy will have attached itself all over you and not just from the neck downwards.

After you've dried yourself, don't put back on any of the clothes you've just removed. Place them in the laundry bin, and instead put on something clean and loose that you enjoy wearing.

. . . .

And this one will help you to 'peel off' any energy impurities that have attached themselves to you during the day.

CLEARING THE COBWEBS

Sit next to the running tap water. Imagine that your body is covered in a fine cobweb. Lightly touch yourself as you imagine removing the cobweb by wiping it off with your hands, working over every part of your body in turn. Your physical hand actions must match your imagined ones. As you do this, frequently hold your hands under running water to rid yourself of the energy you're removing. Don't forget to remove the cobwebby energy from your back, the nape of your neck, the palms of your hands and the soles of your feet.

You may want to change this exercise if you have a fear of spiders and don't like the thought of cobwebs. Imagine that, instead of a cobweb, you're covered in a fine film of dust that you've got to remove.

. . . .

I love the following meditation. You may particularly enjoy it if you're strongly attuned to the water element. It's great for express clearing after your energy has become 'dirty'.

THE WHIRLPOOL

Choose a time when you won't be disturbed and can fully engage with this meditation.

Intention: to burn off any negative energy that you've picked up.

1. Imagine that one current of water enters your body through your crown and another enters from your feet. They meet in your abdomen, in the space between your navel and solar plexus chakras, and join to create a whirlpool of salty seawater.

2. Ask the salt in the water to absorb any negative energy that you've acquired and to take away everything negative inside you.

3. When you know that the salt water has absorbed all the negativity inside you, imagine that you're floating on the calm waters of the sea, feeling completely at peace.

4. While you're imagining this you can physically sway your body, as if you are being gently swirled around by the sea.

5. Do this for as long as it's comfortable. When you feel lighter and cleaner, slowly bring your awareness back to the room. Don't drain the water.

Cleaning as a Spiritual Ritual

The next time you're dusting or putting things in order in your home, treat the process like a spiritual ritual. Make it a symbolic act as well as a physical task, so you're investing your spiritual forces in it. The external affects the internal.

When tidying up, try to involve your eyes, ears, hands and even your breathing as you connect with the different areas of the room. Look at the objects you're cleaning or tidying up, and really engage with them rather than going through the motions on autopilot while thinking of something else entirely.

You don't need to do this every time you clean your house, but doing it every now and then is a wonderful way to honour your home and make tidying it part of a meditation. Just as some people never compromise about putting lots of effort and intention into treating their physical body as a temple for their energy, so you should not shy away from spending time and physical effort on cleaning your home and truly connecting with it. It will be worth it, because your home will become your sanctuary.

CLEANSING THE ENERGY OF YOUR HOME

This exercise features the very potent combination of visualization and physical activity for maximum impact. Choose a time when you won't be disturbed or interrupted. Switch off your phone, sit down and spend a few minutes relaxing.

Intention: cleansing the energy of your home using the power of your mind.

1. In your mind's eye, picture your home and see yourself ('Create Your Energy Twin' on p.154 might help with this) entering the first room. See yourself standing in the middle of the room. Take time to tune in to the energy around you and gain a sense of the space.

2. Now imagine putting your hand in your pocket and pulling out a handful of gold dust. Open your hand and blow the gold dust into the room. You can become a physical part of this visualization by actually puffing on your outstretched hand as you imagine blowing the gold dust into the room. It is sparkling and shimmering, and it completely fills the entire room. The inside of the room is now shimmering with gold dust.

3. Picture the gold dust filling every corner, every nook and cranny, and don't leave the room until this has happened. Try to imagine this as vividly as you can, to increase the effectiveness of the exercise.

4. When the room is completely full of gold dust, you can leave it and move on to the next one, where you repeat the entire process. Work around your home in this way until you have cleansed every single room. If you have walk-in cupboards or wardrobes, make sure that you cleanse these in the same way.

. . . .

CHAPTER 13

Dealing with Energy Vampires

In Chapter 7, Auric 'Fungi', we looked at energy vampires – people who feed off the energy of others in a parasitic way. And as I explained there, it's very important that we all recognize our *own* tendencies towards energy vampirism. Doing so will enable us to own our energy more effectively and take personal responsibility for ourselves and our behaviour.

It can be very tempting to tell ourselves that we're the good ones and that we need to be wary of external forces – but that's not how it works. We all encounter situations in which we could slip into becoming an energy vampire, even if it's short-lived. It's not a case of being perfect while everyone else is in the wrong, or acting like a spiritual snob.

Breaking the Vampire–Donor Connection

Are you locked into a long-term connection with an energy vampire? Becoming aware of this is one thing, but you also need to know what to do about it. The best way to start is by asking yourself some honest questions and not judging the answers that come to you.

Ask yourself *how* you're investing in your relationship with this person. What's the deal? Do you want to please them, and will you therefore put up with them draining your energy? Are they useful to you? Do you feel guilty about them for some reason? Or maybe you feel sorry for them? How do you hope the relationship will benefit you?

Unfortunately, the sad truth is that you won't get *any* benefit from this relationship. Donating your energy to an energy vampire will never lead to anything that will serve you, and it may prevent you from living an authentic life. Remember: if you don't own your energy you're donating it to someone else. Maybe you're placing yourself in an imaginary hierarchy and willingly becoming someone's energy slave? If you don't alter that connection, the result will be a life-long sentence of energy deficiency for you.

It can take time for you to understand exactly what's happening in your dealings with an energy vampire, so be patient and keep questioning yourself. It's really important to do this, or you won't break the donor–vampire connection. You can practise lots of exercises to protect yourself from the energy vampire in your life, but they won't make any difference if you're running an inner programme that says you'll benefit from your relationship with them.

This 'energy donation through vampirism' is never an investment: it's always a loss, even if you do hope it will turn into something. It's energy acquired through abuse and it will never serve you. If you struggle to address this issue, in my mind it's best to see a psychologist. Energy healing alone won't fix it, so please take a holistic approach.

How to Avoid Being an Energy Vampire

We've all done it – after a terrible day at work, we've gone home and taken out our frustration on our partner or our children. Or we've felt exhausted on our way to see a friend, and once we were with them, we used their energy to perk ourselves up.

So it's important to think about the state of your energy before you make contact with others, whether it's face to face, in a phone call, online or in any other way. You must protect your personal space but also be careful that you don't pollute and damage other people's space. This is all part of living authentically. We need to be aware of the way we're living and of our inner balance, and we must also protect the inner balance of the people around us.

Stabilize Your Energy

Since ancient times, spiritual masters have believed that the world is composed of the four basic elements of fire, earth, air and water. These energetic forces of nature were viewed as governing parts of the Universe and everything in it, including humans. It was said that all four of these forces must be balanced so that the fifth spiritual element of ether, known as *prana* in India, or as I like to call it, the life force, can manifest itself.

The next time you're feeling deflated and are tempted to use someone as your energy charger, or you're venting negativity and trying to treat others as a rubbish bin for your bad day, try stabilizing yourself in a healthy way by using the following tools, which harness the qualities of fire, earth, air and water.

In the same way that you'd reach for a broom immediately after making a mess in the home, you can use these elemental tools as a form of energy hygiene for yourself and your environment. You can also use them as first aid immediately after a negative energy exchange (see Chapter 12).

Intention: to stabilize and clear your energy in order to prevent yourself from becoming an energy vampire.

Step 1: Find Your Element

First of all, choose the element that resonates most strongly with you at the moment. We all have one dominant element within ourselves, and you can use the questions below to establish which is yours. Please note that your resonance with the elements can change throughout your life, so don't automatically choose one without considering the others too.

Fire

❖ Are you enthusiastic, optimistic and passionate?

❖ Do you love gazing into an open fire?

❖ Do you enjoy basking in full sunshine and always turn up the central heating?

Earth

❖ Are you grounded, stable and full of common sense?

❖ Do you love being surrounded by nature?

❖ Do you like gardening or working with wood?

Air

❖ Are you a dreamer, a visionary or a thinker?

❖ Do you find it invigorating to stand in a strong wind?

❖ Do you love being out in the fresh air, or do you always keep your windows open because that way you feel you can breathe?

Water

❖ Are you easily swayed by your emotions or intuition?

❖ Do you love being beside a river or the sea?

❖ Are you affected by the phases of the Moon?

❖ Do you enjoy soaking in a bath?

Step 2: Use Your Element as a Stabilizer

Each element possesses unique properties and characteristics, and I recommend utilizing these as effective, practical tools to balance your energy, as described below.

Fire

Immediately after being exposed to toxic energy, light an open fire (if you have one) and sit next to it while you meditate on the flames. Alternatively, you can light a candle and meditate while looking at the burning flame.

If you know exactly what's draining your energy or making you feed off other people's energy, write it down in detail on a sheet of paper. Now place the paper in the fireplace or a metal bucket and set light to it with a match. Watch as it burns – almost as an act of meditation – until only ashes are left.

Charcoal tablets are also useful for this purpose because they smoke when lit. Place a couple in the top of an essential oil burner, or an old dish or saucer, and set light to them. If you wish, you can add a sprig of dried sage to each one, so it 'smudges' the atmosphere as the charcoal tablet burns.

Finally, here's a very simple but effective meditative exercise that you can do anywhere. Feel your pulse by placing the tips of your right hand on your left wrist, just below the base of your thumb. You'll know you've found the right spot when you can feel your pulse throbbing. Sit calmly and think about the warm blood rushing through your body, filling you with its life-giving energy. Just rest for a while on the waves of your pulse. This is also a great exercise to practise if you feel that the energy of your environment is threatening your unique frequency.

Earth

Immediately following a negative exchange, go into the garden, if you have one, and do some gardening. Instead of wearing protective gloves, let your skin connect with the soil. It will absorb any negative energies and you'll soon feel grounded and peaceful.

Try some barefoot walking. Ideally, you should do this outside, on a patch of grass. If that's not possible, walk around barefoot indoors, especially if you have wooden floors.

How about hugging a tree? If there's one in your garden, wrap your arms around it, so that your energy begins to resonate with that of the tree. You can do this in a park or a wood if you prefer. If you feel self-conscious about hugging a tree in public, sit so close to it that your spine, from your coccyx to the top of your neck, is in contact with its bark.

Air

If you resonate with the element of air, you can do 3-3-3 breathing to reset your energy after an energy attack. All you need to do is inhale through your nose to the count of three, hold your breath to the count of three and then exhale through your mouth to the count of three. Do this for a couple of minutes at a time. When you inhale, try to expand your ribcage sideways, almost as though it's an accordion; and when you exhale, do it through your mouth, and almost as though you're sighing.

After a heated argument or a tough meeting, open the windows in the room and allow the outside air to flood in. This is even better if a gentle breeze is blowing. Let the movement of air blow away your own negative energy and clean the energy of the room at the same time.

Not everyone enjoys or tolerates the scent of joss sticks, but if you do you can light one and let it gently clean the air around you. Frankincense is perfect, whether you burn it as incense or use a few pieces of frankincense resin, because it disperses clusters of negative energy and increases your breathing capacity.

If you're lucky enough to live in the country, go outside when it's breezy and surrender to the wind. Let it blow through your hair. Open your arms and become almost part of that blowing wind.

Water

Immediately after a conflict, or when you're feeling drained by others, go for a swim or sit beside some running water, such as a stream or river, or simply a running tap. Imagine that all your attached negative energy is being swept away by the current of the water; and that you're synchronizing with the sound of running water.

Another great option is to take a shower. The temperature of the water doesn't matter, so you can have it as cold or as hot as you want. What you must do, though, is ensure that the water cascades over the crown of your head downwards, so it takes all the toxic energy away with it. You'll need a large volume of water for this exercise, so tip a large bowl or bucket of water over your head if your showerhead is small. Engage with the water and hold to your intention of cleansing. In your mind, ask the water to absorb and wash away all the negative energy that you've accumulated.

If it's not convenient for you to take a shower, you can fill a sink or large bowl with water. Cup both hands, scoop up the water and splash your face with it. Keep scooping, and allow the water to run down your face until you feel lighter. Pat your face dry with a clean towel.

If you're short of time but need instant help, you can mindfully drink a glass of water. Fill a glass with water that's slightly cooler than the temperature of the room. Sit down and relax, slowly sip the water, and mentally follow its path as it travels down your oesophagus into your stomach. Be really mindful of how the water travels through your chest. Finish drinking the glass of water and keep observing the sensations left by the flowing water. This is a helpful and quick way of recalibrating your energy when you're at work.

Make some crystal water. Buy a clear glass atomizer, place some small pieces of crystal in it – those that resonate most powerfully with water are amethyst and aquamarine – and fill it with water. Place the atomiser on a sunny windowsill, so the Sun's rays can penetrate it. Leave it there for several hours, after which it'll be ready for use.

Spray your personal space liberally with the crystal water whenever you feel you're about to switch to an energy vampire state, and it will help to prevent it from happening. When your atomiser is empty, tip out the crystals, rinse them and the bottle thoroughly under a running tap and then refill it using the same method as before.

Part VI

PRACTISING
SAFE
LIVING

CHAPTER 14

Energy Prophylactics

The word 'prophylactic' comes from the Greek for 'to guard by taking advance measures', and it usually refers to the prevention of physical disease. However, in this chapter we'll be using it in the sense of focusing on safeguarding the aura and other aspects of energy hygiene.

Sadly, too many people address their wellness only *after* a problem has occurred, so the approach immediately becomes remedial and therapeutic. If you want to own your energy and stop the endless cycle of winning it back from disease, auric prophylactics and energy hygiene in general should become part of your lifestyle. This is the key to sustainable wellness!

My principles of energy prophylactics have two main pillars:

❖ A resilient aura

❖ Authentic personal vibrations

You already know that when your aura is balanced, its outer layer, the auric skin, acts as your best protector, provided by nature itself.

The auric skin has a rubber-like quality and it repels toxic or harmful energy. So, in order to improve the elasticity of your auric skin you have to harmonize and nourish your aura – your strong and buoyant energy field will plump it up from within.

According to the Law of Vibration and the Law of Resonance, which I described in Part 2, the type of energy you attract very much depends on the vibrations you're broadcasting and on your vibrational 'radius'. In other words, when your aura's vibrational signal is strong and clear, like a ship's sonar, it will navigate through the surrounding sea of energy waves so you can attract and connect only with what is uplifting and beneficial to you.

So, now, let me show you how you can boost your aura and amplify your personal vibrations.

How to Enhance Your Aura

In the modern Western world, a balanced and well-nourished aura is becoming a precious and sought-after commodity. We're feeling so overwhelmed by life and overexposed to our environment that we're instinctively trying to create a buffer for our inner space. However, in the absence of the right tools to do so, we're resorting to desperate measures, such as telling loved ones to leave us alone when we're busy, sabotaging loving relationships, wearing headphones when at home or outside, or running off to faraway lands.

Please be aware that this kind of detachment and defensiveness will never lead to the creation of your aura or a sense of inner space. It will always be an illusion as temporary as sticking plaster, which the force of the energies around you will keep stripping away from your soul. Our aura is not the equivalent of a bubble of isolation, as we discussed earlier in the book. Stay open but assertive with the help of healthy personal boundaries and self-awareness.

Why Are Boundaries So Important?

Have you ever calculated how many seconds there are in a year? The answer is 31,536,000, which sounds like a massive amount, but it soon shrinks when you subtract the number of seconds you spend eating, sleeping, working and all the other dutiful activities that form part of your daily routine.

Even if we live to the age of 80, the time we devote to fulfilling our passions in life will usually only add up to seven or eight years. We have to remember that life is very short, and we must be very careful with our precious time. This fact should make us more assertive about guarding our personal space, creating strong personal boundaries, and living an authentic life. Otherwise, we might find that we've spent those seven or eight years focusing our energy on something or someone that has no relevance to our true self at all. What a waste of life!

Establish Your Boundaries

If you don't know what your boundaries are, other people won't either. So it's very important for all of us to create strong boundaries and stick to them.

❖ Decide which are the most important boundaries for you, and write them down on a sheet of paper that you can pin up in a prominent place, to remind you of your 'rules'. Here are some examples: *Go to bed at 10pm every night; no working on weekends; don't engage in gossip.* Share your boundaries with the people in your life.

❖ 'Do not speak unless it improves on silence' is one of my favourite Buddhist sayings. Only participate in conversations and activities that resonate with you or uplift you. You can, of course, compromise, but only as a personal decision rather than as a response to manipulation.

❖ Prevent people from being intrusive – for example, by offering you unwanted advice, asking you intimate questions or generally being uncomfortably nosy.

❖ Spend your free time with people you feel at ease with; those who inspire you; and those with whom you have a common interest. Go back to Part 2 to refresh your memory on filtering your social circle.

❖ Always ask permission before imposing on someone's personal space and expect the same from others. This request shouldn't come from a cold place of egotistical arrogance but from a warm place of kindness and self-love.

❖ Practise self-respect by embracing your individual rights. 'No' is a full sentence. You don't have to justify anything to anyone if something feels wrong to you, or if you feel intruded upon. No one should manipulate you into putting others' needs before your own. You may choose to do this, but you should never be forced into it. Never do anything out of guilt.

❖ Low self-worth is the most common emotion to dismantle your boundaries; so try to practise the navel chakra affirmation 'I deserve' every day. Your boundaries aren't a self-indulgent, frivolous luxury but a basic human necessity and part of your natural mechanism of self-preservation.

❖ Let your behaviour, rather than your words, speak for you. People will be more inclined to violate your boundaries if your actions, your body language and the energy of your words aren't aligned.

❖ Your boundaries shouldn't turn your aura into a bunker and you into a fear-driven recluse. Stay open to life and address any psychological traumas in your past so you can snap out of hiding-in-defence mode.

❖ Stop assuming responsibility for everyone. Your personal boundaries will be nonexistent if you 'carry' too many people.

❖ No one can tell you what your limits are. Only you can set these for yourself. Rely only on your own intuition as a barometer. For example, only you will know whether one glass of wine is enough for you or whether you can tolerate half a bottle.

❖ Look after your home. As a healer, I've observed that if we disconnect from our living space or fill it with material or energetic clutter we tend to compromise our boundaries. Besides, as you know, it also creates a breeding ground for energy 'fungi'.

❖ Live mindfully so you can really connect to the world around you and not live on autopilot. Use your daily activities as an opportunity for meditation by really focusing on what you're doing and screening out all distractions – try this as you dry yourself after a shower, on your walk to work, or as you perform any of the other tasks you do each day. Connect with all of your senses to what you're doing and what's around you. This will enable you to be fully aware, assertive and in control of your environment. You'll also be activating your Sushumna meridian of now.

❖ Learn to feel comfortable in your own skin. Take the time to connect with the temple of your physical body in a mindful way – whether you're applying body lotion, preparing food or putting on your shoes. Connecting fully with what you're doing is healthy for your body and it will induce the feeling of being comfortable in your own skin.

Amplify this sense by tuning in more carefully to your emotions. How does your emotional climate change throughout the day? Which emotions and sensations are you experiencing in your body? When you open the fridge door to look for something to eat, is it really because you're hungry? Maybe you don't need that slice of cheese and instead need to acknowledge that you're feeling angry about something, or anxious about your child; or maybe you simply feel bored and need a distraction. Your personal boundaries will be so much stronger with the application of self-reflective awareness.

❖ Stop trying to be nice to everyone.

❖ Learn to receive. A state of gratitude and appreciation is vital for our boundaries and our aura in general. It shifts our focus from the negative towards the positive. This will prevent you from searching for and 'hooking' toxic energy. Instead you'll be recognizing, validating and appreciating positivity in your life, and in doing so you'll be attracting even more of it. Besides, this also primes your auric skin to absorb even more positivity and for your auric sonar to register an ever wider sweep of positive waves.

Control Your Inner Weather

Your aura thrives not only when you create healthy boundaries but also when you control and honour your inner rhythms. You're probably already aware of the way that negative emotions and distracting thoughts disconnect you from your inner calm and at times make you feel as if you're in the eye of a storm. I hope the insights I've shared throughout the book will help you to master your emotional, mental and energetic reactions.

Now, though, I'd like to mention two of the biological and physiological triggers that can lead you to over-react, sabotage your inner energy flow and destabilize your aura:

❖ An over-reactive amygdala

❖ Disturbed circadian rhythms

These factors are often overlooked by people who focus *only* on the metaphysical tools for stabilizing their aura, which explains why so many of us live in a state of inner volatility. We must engage with and fine-tune our physical body when balancing our aura. Let's take a look at these triggers.

The Over-Reactive Amygdala

The amygdala is a tiny part of the brain that can be described as the emotional 'alarm clock' of the body. It conducts our biological response to fears about the present and, crucially, about things that occurred in the past. So many of us are stuck in a 'negative gear' and are unable to tell the difference between negative events from the past and what's happening to us now. This leads to a chronic tendency to project past negativity onto the present.

When our negative thoughts are always dominant, our amygdala becomes overactive and hyper-vigilant, thereby activating our nervous and hormonal systems, which in turn create the habit of over-reaction. We often talk about fear and anxiety as though they're interchangeable states of mind, but they aren't. Fear is our reaction to actual danger, whereas anxiety is our reaction to what we perceive is dangerous.

An over-reactive amygdala will make you needlessly paranoid about energy vampires and many other violations of your energy, and your brain will continue to provide neurological support for your negative mindset. You can think of an unbalanced amygdala as like a faulty burglar alarm that's always going off because it sees everything as a threat.

Interestingly, the amygdala not only triggers the fight-or-flight response that's so often associated with fear, but also the freeze response. I often encounter patients who are in a 'comfortably numb' state. They aren't running away from a problem and neither are they confronting it. Instead, they're almost freezing up or disassociating themselves from the present. From an energy point of view, their aura is almost trying to disappear rather than face up to the reality of what they need to deal with.

This is a hugely exhausting state to be in, and it requires a complex therapeutic approach if the patient is to feel alive and alert again. Sadly, many people adapt to this 'frozen' state and accept it as perfectly normal.

Don't forget that the amygdala is always on the lookout for danger, whether the threat is real or perceived, so it can trigger a survival response. That's why, once again, it's important to cultivate a healthier, more neutral perception of reality rather than jumping into a kneejerk, negative attitude.

Retrain Your Amygdala

Your amygdala should not own your energy, *you* should! Luckily, there are steps you can take to retrain this part of your brain so it can release its grip:

❖ Hit the 'pause button' before you react to anything by cultivating the 'observer state' I described in Chapter 11. The meditations *The Neutral State* and *The Periscope* are very beneficial for learning to adopt a more balanced attitude.

❖ Own your moments by staying present through mindfulness and connecting to the energy of now.

❖ Nourish your amygdala by doing things that make you happy. When you truly connect and stay with an activity that gives you pleasure and joy, even if it's only for 30 seconds, this helps to rewire and regulate the amygdala. Whenever possible, try to stay connected with sensual pleasures, and really absorb them – whether that's smelling a beautiful rose, stroking your child's hair, watching a bee buzzing around your garden, or anything else that makes you smile.

❖ Use daily affirmations to programme your mind for balanced perception and positive attitudes.

❖ Eat a high-quality diet rich in vitamins D, B6, B3 and C and in L-theanine, GABA, magnesium, zinc and Omega 3. Serotonin, the neurotransmitter that induces happiness and wellbeing, is produced in the gut so probiotics, too, are very important for boosting our overall mood.

Disturbed Circadian Rhythms

Our circadian rhythms (or biological clock) regulate our asleep–awake state, digestive system and the secretion of hormones. They also help us to adapt to changes in our environment.

When you're leading a chaotic lifestyle you destabilize your body's circadian rhythms, which also sabotages the balanced harmony of your vibrations. You lose the beauty of your inner melody. Remember that your physical body is the visible layer of your aura, so regulating the rhythms of this layer will help to harmonize the others too.

Balance Your Circadian Rhythms

Here are some things you can do to support and balance your circadian rhythms:

❖ Maintain regular times for going to bed and getting up

❖ Minimize your exposure to artificial light, especially the blue light of digital screens, at night

❖ Limit artificial stimulants such as coffee

❖ Be mindful while eating, and focus on chewing

Your Authentic Vibrations

The title of this book features two key words: 'own' and 'your'. In order to amplify your vibrations, you need first of all to calibrate *who you are*. Only *authentic* personal vibrations can create a strong and positive frequency for your energy field, your aura, and manifest what is *yours*.

Michelangelo once reflected on one of his famous masterpieces: 'David was already in the marble … I just took away everything that wasn't him.' I adopt the same attitude when working with energy. We just need to reveal what's already there because in essence we're all beings of light with a unique imprint.

Let's begin by getting to know ourselves in the best way we can. Each of us has to learn what's most important to us, what our values are, and discover every other aspect of our personality. We must be prepared to be intimate with ourselves – really connecting with our true self – even if we don't always like what we see. If this concept is new to you, because you've never really had an intimate connection with your true self, then you'll have to start with baby steps.

Discover Your Energy ID

What is the signature of your life force? As you know, everyone's energy has a unique frequency, so mine will be different from yours. The differences don't matter. What's important is that when we live beautifully and well, we live authentically.

Your Aura's Potential (Size) + Your Unique Frequency + Your Authentic Vibration = Your Energy ID

We have to be mindful of our energy ID. When someone is clean, they smell good, and when they are authentic in their energy we experience them as being full of light. We feel better for being with them. We know that these people have clear energy because even if we can't see it we can *sense* it. In Russia, we talk about someone being 'a clear person' – just as the English phrase 'clear sky' means that it's free of clouds.

The following exercises will help you to discover and understand your unique energy ID. Please note that revealing your aura's potential and refining your authentic frequency is a lifelong task. I tend to view it not as a job done once, but as a continuous journey of self-discovery. Your intuition will let you know if you are on the right path.

YOUR INNER PECKING ORDER

What's the 'pecking order' in your life? You can have fun with this, picturing a chicken's roosting perch, with five parallel bars rising upwards from the floor. The highest bar represents your top priorities in life, and you're sitting on that bar. Where do you place your needs on the bars beneath you?

. . . .

This next exercise will help you to identify your core values and beliefs.

DISCOVER YOUR CORE BELIEFS

Choose a time when you won't be disturbed. Switch off your phone and all other distractions. You'll need a sheet of paper and a pen or pencil; don't use your phone or a computer.

Intention: to help you maintain a strong self-image and a strong sense of identity.

1. Sit calmly and breathe slowly. Meditate on what is most valuable and most important in your life. This may be only one thing or person, or it might be several.

2. Write down the thoughts that come to you without editing or judging them. Just let your ideas flow.

3. When you've finished, leave the sheet of paper in a prominent position, such as on your desk, fridge or in the bathroom, so you see it several times each day. In this way, you'll continually be reminded of your values, beliefs and priorities in life.

. . . .

When completing the following exercise, you can add more questions that are relevant to the life you lead.

WHAT MAKES YOU DIFFERENT?

Sit quietly with a notebook and a pen (not an electronic device) in a place where you won't be interrupted. Consider the following questions and write down your answers.

Intention: to discover and celebrate what makes you unique.

✧ What makes you unique?

✧ How do you differ from your parents?

✧ How do you differ from your siblings?

✧ How do you differ from your partner?

✧ How do you differ from your best friends?

✧ How do you differ from your colleagues?

✧ How different are you from the labels that people apply to you?

✧ How different are you from the nicknames you're given?

✧ How different are you from the rules and ideas that have been imposed on you by your background?

You may not be able to answer each question fully at first. Let the ideas come, and be prepared to add to them whenever another answer occurs to you. Gradually, you'll be able to build up a strong picture of your unique energy ID.

WHAT MAKES YOUR LIFE GOOD?

Set aside some time for yourself and sit quietly, with a notebook and pen by your side.

Intention: to remind yourself of what makes you happy.

1.   Think about all the things that make your life good. Focus on the activities you enjoy and write them down. Leave plenty of space between each item on the list.

2.   Now think about the first activity you've listed and write down all the things you enjoy about it. Then move on to the second activity, and so on until you've worked through the list.

3.   Jot down more activities that occur to you, and describe why you like them.

4.   Now look at all the activities. Do they have key ingredients in common, such as spending time with other people, being creative, or being alone? If you can identify these key ingredients you'll be able to seek more activities that offer them.

For this next exercise you'll need a big folder or box file. Instead of reusing an old one or making do with something tatty, consider buying a special one that you love looking at, so you feel good every time you see it.

YOUR ACHIEVEMENTS FOLDER

Intention: to remind yourself of the success that comes when you're proactive, and to honour your achievements.

✧ Start collecting evidence of all the things you've achieved in your life and put it in the folder or box file. This can be anything and everything that you feel good about, from exam certificates to photos of you doing something you're proud of. These achievements don't have to be what others have praised you for – they can be things that you feel proud of and regard as accomplishments.

✧ If you don't have any physical evidence of an accomplishment or achievement, write it on a piece of paper or card and put it in the folder. For instance, you might want to write about being a good parent or about the time you prevented someone being assaulted.

✧ Include achievements that involved acting on your instincts and intuition, and being fluid with your decisions, rather than just doing what others expected from you.

VIP Versus VAP

In recent years there's been an exciting shift in attitude towards our aspirations, motivations, goals and life in general. Wellness is becoming a new way to be rich, kindness is the new cool, and fulfilment is the new success. And I believe that *authenticity* must become our new wealth.

Hunting for status at work or in society, in order that one can be treated better than anyone else, is becoming a dated aspiration in the modern world. Being a very important person (VIP) might seem attractive but it only highlights an individual's status and essentially, it's a means of validation through impressing others.

It's a concept that's been exploited by the service industry, which extorts money from us by flattering our ego. Someone may be convinced that they've made it in life because they own a yacht, sit in the royal box at the theatre and own multiple homes, but I'd argue that they cannot consider themselves wealthy or an achiever if they don't own their energy.

I want to clarify here that I've absolutely nothing against financial wealth, fame or work status. They deserve to be celebrated! For me, as a healer, there's only one question I would ask: *What was your driver to achieve that and the price tag it carried for your life force?* If you were driven by a desire for fulfilment based on your true values, soul honesty, and authenticity, then, as they say in France, *chapeau* (respect!)

Ultimately, though, I believe that our focus should shift from being a VIP to a VAP – a *very authentic person*. Being a VAP isn't about snobbery, acquiring possessions or striving to be better than others but simply being the best version of ourselves. We're already seeing that more and more people are shifting their aspirations from success to fulfilment and from material possessions to spiritual experiences.

Flashy parties and hedonistic holidays, designed to show off our wealth and intoxicate our bodies, are being replaced by wellness activities and better self-care. Generic living, wellness and healthcare are being transformed by the unprecedented demands for artisan and bespoke experiences.

A VAP isn't interested in how others perceive them – they are concerned only with the attitude they have towards themselves and their relationship with Self. A VAP isn't discriminatory. We *all* can and should be a VAP. It doesn't depend on our status. It's not about what we own, who we know, or how much money we have in the bank. It's about who we truly are. It's possibly the most exclusive club you can join because membership isn't up for sale: you only acquire it through commitment to the authenticity and ownership of your energy. The loud and clear vibrations of your unique energy ID are your membership card.

The VAP Lifestyle

Being a VAP means living in harmony with yourself as well as with the outside world. It also means refusing to waste energy on toxic people or shallow gatherings. When you're a VAP you don't get caught up in emotionally dwelling on the past, and you don't go into self-pity mode when things go wrong. Instead, you sort out your problems as constructively as possible and always do your best to help others.

A VAP isn't ruled by the energy of poverty, so you don't tell yourself that you're not worthy of receiving or utilizing the best you have. You eat high-quality, healthy food and use organic natural products, because as a VAP you take responsibility for your life and health. You care about where the products you buy come from because you also care about the world, nature and your local community.

You generate your own energy and don't use other people's energy to give yourself a boost. You're in the flow. As a VAP you don't have a consumer mindset; instead, you're looking for partners to accompany you through life, rather than paying someone to do everything for you. You live an authentic life according to your own instincts and impulses; you don't copy anyone else; and you have clear boundaries for your personal space and serenity. You're an authority in your world and not a confused jumble of inner fears, limitations and social conditioning. However, at the same time you're someone who lives with humility and humbleness.

As a VAP, hobbies are also important to you, but you choose pastimes that are truly reflective of what you enjoy, rather than because they're fashionable or intended to impress other people. You also create a chemistry with your life, so you live with a sparkle – not only in your eyes but also in your aura.

Spiritual Snobbery

We need to grasp the concept of being a power and an authority in our own personal space without kick-starting our ego and placing ourselves above the natural world and other people. So there must be a balance. Snobbery should be a thing of the past. The energy that you emanate will speak much more loudly than the things you possess. However, please note that it's only the energy of the ego that shouts; the energy of the authentic core speaks in a gentle tone, not an overpowering one.

We should also stop being spiritual snobs; for example, when in a yoga class glancing condescendingly at the beginners while doing our perfectly performed asana, or ridiculing people for not being sufficiently 'evolved' to grasp some insight or other. Life isn't a competition and we really don't *want* to compete with each other in our spirituality. We're all a work in progress.

Besides, the spiritual snob only climbs the ladder of the ego, which disguises itself as spiritual evolution. What a waste of energy!

The Mask

We willingly become energy donors whenever we try to impress other people or bend over backwards in order to fit in – expending our energy for the sake of someone's acceptance. In this instance, and generally each time we deny ourselves permission to be our true self, we cause significant interference and distortion in the flow of our authentic life force. So our inner energy and personality almost become counterfeit – an *imitation* of who we're pretending to be rather than who we really are. Yes, of course we need to be flexible and willing and able to compromise, but we need to avoid breaking ourselves in the process.

The American writer John Updike said that 'celebrity is a mask that eats into your face'. I would like to paraphrase this: we adopt a persona that we hope makes us more popular or more impressive, but it ends up eating into our true face and we start to identify with our 'mask'. In effect, we stop owning our energy while trying to latch onto the energy of our pretend self. This is the most expensive mask you can ever acquire as will cost you dearly in the currency of your life force.

When you're a VAP you don't resort to the 'mask' but honour and accept your 'true face' instead. We all need to learn about living without a mask. In the beginning you might find yourself feeling almost naked and exposed without it, but please resist the temptation to put it back on! The more you own your energy, the less you'll feel the need for a mask.

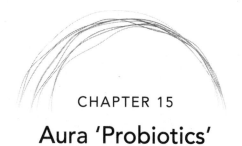

CHAPTER 15

Aura 'Probiotics'

Supplements of probiotics, living organisms found in certain foods, are becoming increasingly popular as a means of supporting and enhancing the natural microflora, or bacteria, in our digestive system. The inner flora of our vibrations also require 'probiotics' in order to thrive and adapt to changes.

You won't find these special 'probiotics' in any shop – they are something you can generate yourself by using the tremendous power of your imagination and your mind. My formula for them is:

Intention + Inspiration + Gratitude = Aura 'Probiotics'

Your aura won't be able to blossom without these components. You can invest in and connect to various sources of energy but if you and your life are lacking intention, inspiration and gratitude, you're unlikely to flourish.

❖ Using the power of your mind to create an *intention* will form a 'vibration template' for the outcome you desire, so both your energy and Universal energy can flow towards it.

❖ The high-frequency state of *gratitude* anchors you in a state of appreciation for what you already have and for the gift of life itself. It prevents you from disowning your present and turns you aura into a magnet for positive energy.

❖ *Inspiration* is a state of alignment with your spirit – it's your internal spark and an uplifting wave that you generate through the chemistry between your authentic core and the stimuli in your environment.

When you're inspired you feel fire in your solar plexus chakra. You feel a call to action for what you believe and you stand tall in your authenticity. I hope that, throughout this book, I've helped to ignite your spirit by inspiring you to align with your aura and your inner truth. Now, I'd like to share a little more about the power of your intention so you can create the best blueprint for your life.

Intention: Your Spiritual Laser

In Russia, we say there is no favourable wind when you don't have a direction. It's so important to formulate a direction in life, so your energy and the Universe can conspire to help you.

Intention can be viewed as a positive common vector or, as I call it, a spiritual laser. For me as a healer, intention is a template of your destination, which also helps you to create a groove in which your energy and Universal energy can flow and carry you towards it. The most simple and common example of intention is a positive affirmation, as this makes a statement which then moulds your energy to back it up.

Try to spend some time figuring out what your desired destination and outcome are. Many people lack this focus and as a result they disperse their energy too widely. Their spiritual laser isn't powerful enough to cut through the groove in the field of energies and templates that surround us all and inhabit our inner space. This can also explain why we might not be moving forward in life.

It's important to ask yourself questions about your intention, so you can be absolutely certain that you're seeking something you really need. This means being very honest with yourself about what's behind your intention. For example, you might think you're looking for love when what you're really doing is trying to escape a feeling of loneliness. Intention must be based on, and reflect, your truth, otherwise it won't carry any potency.

I'm not saying this is easy! It can take enormous courage and humility to be honest with yourself about your true intentions. And it may also take time before you become aware of what your real intentions are. We often hide behind false ideas or excuses, or even fairy tales (such as 'My life will be perfect when I find the man/woman/job of my dreams' or 'when I lose weight'), and these become such a strong part of ourselves that we completely believe them.

However, these false ideas and narratives come from our 'inner troll', not from our authentic core. As we discussed earlier, our 'inner troll' isn't invested in us thriving. It feeds off negative vibrations and it won't help us to acquire more light because that's the last thing it wants. So, please, pay attention to the part of yourself that's setting an intention.

You might think that desire and intention are the same things, but they aren't. Desire is a very low-frequency state. It often focuses on instant gratification and the search for a quick fix and, as a result, leads to disillusionment and disappointment. Desire has a strong energy of angst. It's connected to 'I want'. Intention is connected to what we need and to what serves our higher self.

227

The Secret of Creating a Good Intention

When you're sure you have a healthy and positive intention, you need to word it in a way that will bring you the results you're looking for. As I've already explained, it's very important not to include the very thing you want to change but instead to choose positive words and phrases.

You must also look at the bigger picture and not at fragmented areas of your life. For example, if you have back pain and you want it to get better, you should not focus only on the back pain. You should focus on becoming healthy throughout your *entire system*, so it can function wholesomely as nature intended.

It's also really important to choose an intention that will benefit others and not just yourself. This doesn't mean making sacrifices or putting yourself last, but deciding how you can use your newly acquired vibration template to help others or the whole world.

How will you be of service to a higher good? This might be really simple. Let's say you want to improve your energy levels. Your intention is to be full of vitality and energy, which will not only benefit you but also allow you to take better care of your loved ones and to become involved in community volunteering.

Gratitude

We often think of gratitude as simply good manners. However, I'd encourage you to look at it as an all-encompassing emotional, or even spiritual, state of being. Gratitude opens the doors to the spiritual realms.

Gratitude contains the word 'attitude', which should be the default filter through which you look at your life. As a result, your aura will become more attractive: it will not only have a more beautiful glow, it will also gain even more power to attract positive, high-frequency vibrations. As Oprah Winfrey said: 'Be thankful for what you have; you'll end up having more. If you concentrate on what you don't have, you will never, ever have enough.'

Gratitude also neutralizes the toxic effects of the negative energies around you. It will shift your energy towards the Sushumna meridian of now, because when we're not grateful for what we have, we tend to devalue our present. Besides, when you're focusing only on what you lack, according to the Law of Resonance you'll be attracting the low-frequency energy of deficiency.

Therefore, I'd recommend that, when praying or meditating on your intention, you always express gratitude first for what you have and *then* ask for something else, rather than only asking and expecting to receive. Many people fail to attract a better energy and life because it's not possible to be a good magnet if you aren't anchored in the present moment and are concentrating on deficiency. Remember: your focus shapes your reality!

Fortunately we all have the ability and opportunity to cultivate gratitude. Rather than complaining about your problems and circumstances, take a few moments to focus on all that you have. The French novelist Alphonse Karr once said: 'Some people are always grumbling because roses have thorns; I'm thankful that thorns have roses.' Try to reflect on the areas where your life is flowering but you're too blinded by the thorns to notice. The more grateful you are, the more you'll register beautiful and positive things around you. You just need to train your inner 'antenna' to pick up on those things.

I'd recommend that every night before going to sleep you create a 'virtual gratitude journal'. Imagine three positive events that occurred during the day. They don't have to be anything major, just simple moments like feeling the warmth of the Sun on your face while sitting in a traffic jam in your car or receiving a hug from someone you love. The secret is to imagine them as vividly as possible, almost trying to recreate the feeling with all of your senses. I want you to 'wear' each moment again. Then give yourself a big smile and *feel* the gratitude with your entire being.

One of my patients shared with me that she's created a 'jar of gratitude'. She took a big empty jar, decorated it herself and every day she deposits in it small pieces of paper on which she's written three positive occurrences. She loves having this 'bank of positivity' in her home as a constant reminder of her life's silver linings. Don't be afraid to count your blessings!

And every morning before leaving home, put on your invisible 'glasses of positivity'. Make it your choice to have a more balanced, positive outlook on life. Try to commit to the state of appreciation and gratitude, so you don't take the gift of life for granted. You'll discover that the Universe will rhyme with you by sending more beauty and abundance your way.

Part VII

. . . .

YOUR
INSTANT
ENERGY
REBOOT
WITH
ALLA

CHAPTER 16

The 'Energyceutical' Power Meditation: *Own Your Energy*

You and your aura don't need to be fixed: you aren't broken! Your energy could be blocked, confused, damaged or depleted, but not broken. In this book, my focus has not been on mending you, but on helping you unfold, unleash and celebrate your authenticity.

Owning your energy is your birthright, and so I've designed a special meditation to help you reclaim it. I graded this meditation with a new 'energyceutical' category to highlight its ability to saturate maximum auric layers with positive vibrations and boost your life force on the deepest of levels. I also call it a power meditation because during this meditative process you will harness both inbuilt power reserves, and the outer powers of nature to revive your unique frequency.

This isn't a short, quick-fix meditation, so for the rest of this section I'm inviting you to join me on a healing journey. At the end of it, your shining aura and the authentic melody of your soul will provide the grand finale of the book!

You've learned how important the chakras and meridians are for our wellbeing and as tools for self-healing. You're also aware of the structure of the aura and the functions of its layers. The energy vortexes of the chakras are radiating through the first three layers of your aura – the physical, emotional and mental.

The power master meditation uses beautiful, multicoloured sensory visualizations as a healing catalyst for the emotional layer, affirmations for the mental layer, and carefully orchestrated breathing for the physical layer.

You'll be utilizing as many senses as possible during the meditation. Using a combination of imaginary pictures and strong verbal statements will engage both hemispheres of your brain. This will help you to develop a much more balanced perception of the reality around you – something that's crucial for achieving sustainable wellness.

Guidelines for Practising the Meditation

The more often you practise this meditation, the better the results will be. Use it as an essential part of your energy hygiene routine, almost like a shower for your aura!

❖ As with any meditation, it's best to do it before breakfast or at the end of the working day, and ideally not just before going to bed. However, you should listen to your intuition and do it whenever you feel it's the right time.

❖ If you wish, you can record yourself as you read the entire meditation out loud, and then listen to the recording as you practise; or instead you can read one stage at a time from the book, and then practise that stage before moving on to the next one, and so on. Just choose whichever method works best for you.

234

❖ Throughout the meditation, I'd like you to breathe in through your nose and out through your mouth. The outbreath should almost feel like a sigh so, please, relax your entire face, especially your lips.

❖ Before practising, find a place to sit (preferably) or lie where you'll be comfortable but won't fall asleep. Take off any jewellery, wear loose clothes made from natural fibres, let your hair hang loose, and if possible don't wear any make-up. Uncross your arms and legs. Needless to say, your phone must be switched off! This is *your* time – your one-to-one with your soul.

Let's begin.

THE POWER MASTER MEDITATION:
OWN YOUR ENERGY

Start by spending a few minutes focusing on your breath and calming your thoughts. Just rest on the waves of your gentle breathing. Inhale. Hold for a moment while focusing on the centre of your chest. Make your exhalation last a few seconds longer than your inhalation. While you do this, begin to reflect on what you're grateful for in your life, the possessions that you appreciate, and what/who you truly love.

With each breath, your body drops deeper into relaxation. It becomes heavier and heavier, yet at the same time you're sensing that your inner spirit is getting lighter and lighter. Now, plant your intention into this meditation. Say in your mind, 'I choose to reclaim my wholeness. I compose my own inner harmony. I am fully embracing the commitment to my true self. I love and honour my authenticity.'

Now imagine your body is a tree. Roots are growing through your feet, a tree trunk through your spine and neck, and branches are growing through your head. Focus on your feet. The tree's roots are growing deeper and deeper into the ground. You can feel an incredibly strong gravitational pull from the centre of the Earth. This force pulls your roots further and further down towards the core of our planet.

Express heartfelt gratitude to the Earth for the body that your soul inhabits, for your food, all your material possessions, your home, money, survival, all your earthly pleasures. Let your entire body be soaked in this state of appreciation, and radiate love towards our planet. Ask the Earth to accept this energy. Then feel the Earth lovingly answering you by sending a cool blue crystal energy, like a stream of spring water, through the roots of your feet; up through the tree trunk and branches, through your entire body.

Say to yourself, 'I am aligned with the Earth's energy and I allow myself to receive it.' Stay with this feeling. Through your feet, keep drawing from this infinite well of terrestrial energy. Send its fresh, crystal-clear flow higher and higher until you feel it filling your entire being, and visualize it coming out through the top of your head. Enjoy the radiance of the blue light as it glows through your pores with a sensation of spearmint coolness. Ignite the belief that the Earth will always support your courage to live authentically, and trust that it will always meet your true needs.

While still feeling the grounding gravitational pull of terrestrial energy, bring your awareness to the top of your head and visualize once again the beautiful leafy branches growing through your head and stretching towards the sky. See them growing higher and higher, all the way up towards the Sun, planets, stars and the infinite galaxies of the limitless Universe.

Now imagine a bright light emerging from the deepest core of the cosmos. It's getting brighter and brighter as your branches stretch towards it. All the space above you is filled with a bright white light with a golden glow and your leaves are bathing in its warm light.

Now express heartfelt gratitude to the Universe for all the love you have in your life, the people you love and who love you, for your life's lessons, your inspirations, your insights, for being a home for your soul and for the gift of life itself.

Once again I want your entire body to be soaked in this state of appreciation and to radiate love towards the Universe. Ask the Universe to accept this energy, then feel it lovingly answering you by sending warm glowing white light, like a powerful ray of sunshine, through your leaves, down the branches, through the top of your head, through your tree trunk, through your entire body and through your roots.

Say to yourself 'I am aligned with Universal energy and I allow myself to receive it.' Stay with this feeling. Keep drawing this limitless source of Universal energy down through the top of your head until its warm, glowing, feather-soft light fills your entire being. Visualize it coming out through the soles of your feet.

Enjoy the radiance of the shimmering glow coming out through your pores and a sensation of warm, cosy softness within. Ignite the belief that the Universe will always be your abundant source of energy, and trust that you're always loved.

Now, let's coordinate your breathing with your visualizations. Inhale through your nose, as though smelling a flower, and as you do so draw cool blue terrestrial energy upwards through the soles of your feet and all the way out through the top of your head. Exhale through your mouth, drawing the warm, glowing, feather-soft light through the top of your head and out through the soles of your feet.

Breathing in, draw in the energy of the Earth. Breathing out, draw in the energy of the Universe. Keep doing this for a few moments while placing your right hand on your solar plexus and covering it with your left if you're a woman (do the reverse if you're a man). The solar plexus is the centre where you calibrate your unique energy ID from the matrix of terrestrial and Universal energies. Connect to this centre while flushing your aura with the streams of these primal energies.

Now take your awareness into your base chakra, which is at the point between your legs known as the perineum. Imagine that here you ignite a little twinkle of ruby-red light. Focus on your in-breath, imagine the air smells of cinnamon, and draw your breath really deep down into this ball of light. Each time you do so it expands and the glow becomes brighter. The red light creates a pulse of vibrant energy.

Feel this energy. See the light flare and illuminate all the space in and around you with a bright red light. You're inside a bright sparkle of red light. Continue to pay attention to your breathing and now focus on your out-breath. Breathe out as if you're trying to blow out a candle. As you do so, imagine that this out-breath carries with it and away from you any feelings of insecurity; a lack of confidence; dysfunctional routines; rigidity; chaos; and childhood traumas.

Now say, either out loud or in your head: 'I am safe. I am grounded. I accept my body. I take care of the material world I live in.' Take a few gentle breaths while reflecting on how you can create better order in your material life; improve your routines; increase your physical activities; make peace with all your family members; and release the past.

Now move your awareness to the navel chakra, the vitality and sensuality centre. Imagine that here you ignite a little twinkle of orange-gold light. Focus on your in-breath, imagine the air smells of orange blossom, and draw your breath really deep down into this ball of light. Each time you do so it expands and the glow becomes brighter. The orange light creates a pulse of vibrant energy. Feel this energy. See the light flare and illuminate all the space in and around you with a bright orange light. You're inside a bright sparkle of orange light.

Continue to pay attention to your breathing and now focus on your out-breath. Again, breathe out as if you're trying to blow out a candle. As you do so, imagine that the out-breath carries with it and away from you any feelings of worthlessness; being undeserving of goodness; memories of negative past relationships; and limited beliefs about your sexuality and sensuality.

Now say, either out loud or in your head: 'I am the creator of my life. My senses are open and I give myself permission to feel joy. I accept myself. I am enough.' Take a few gentle breaths while reflecting on how you can create more beauty in your life; refine your senses; slow down to appreciate the world around you; spoil yourself and your loved ones more often; and develop more creative or novel ways of doing things.

Then move your awareness to the solar plexus chakra, the centre of personal power, located at the top of your stomach. Imagine that here you ignite a little twinkle of yellow-gold light. Focus on your in-breath, imagine the air smells of lemon, and draw your breath really deep down into this ball of light. Each time you do so it expands and the glow becomes brighter. The yellow light creates a pulse of vibrant energy. Feel this energy. See the light flare and illuminate all the space in and around you with a bright yellow light. You're inside a bright sparkle of yellow light.

Continue to pay attention to your breathing and now focus on your out-breath. As you exhale, imagine that the out-breath carries with it and away from you any feelings of powerlessness; limiting self-beliefs; wrong choices; perfectionism; and people-pleasing tendencies.

Now say, either out loud or in your head: 'I value my uniqueness. I honour my true self. I am aligned with my personal power. My authenticity makes me invincible and allows me to shine.' Take a few gentle breaths while reflecting on your mission in life; where you need to restore your boundaries; what you've accomplished so far; how you feel about your job choices; and your personal step-by-step goals.

Now focus on the centre of your chest, on your heart chakra. Imagine that here you ignite a little twinkle of grass-green light. Focus on your in-breath, imagine the air smells of roses, and draw your breath really deep down into this ball of light. Each time you do so it expands and the glow becomes brighter. The green light creates a pulse of vibrant energy. Feel this energy. See the light flare and illuminate all the space in and around you with a bright, vibrant green light. You're inside a bright sparkle of green light.

Continue to pay attention to your breathing and now focus on your out-breath. As you exhale, imagine that the out-breath carries with it and away from you any feelings that you're unworthy of love; anything that suppresses your emotions; past emotional scars that shut down your heart; cynicism; and old grudges about your parents and your partner.

Now say, either out loud or in your head: 'I am love. I let love in. I invite more compassion into my heart for myself and towards others. I carry less judgement and more kindness. All past hurts are released into the hands of love.' Take a few gentle breaths while reflecting on who you've hurt in your life and to whom you need to apologize; your steps towards self-forgiveness; how you can contribute or volunteer to a charity or your community; how you can be more romantic; and how to be more expressive in your love towards the people who are dear to your heart.

Now move your awareness to your throat chakra, the centre of your honest communication. Imagine that here you ignite a little twinkle of turquoise light. Focus on your in-breath, imagine the air smells of mint, and draw your breath really deep down into this ball of light. Each time you do so it expands and the glow becomes brighter. The turquoise light creates a pulse of vibrant energy. Feel this energy. See the light flare and illuminate all the space in and around you with a bright turquoise light. You're inside a bright sparkle of turquoise light.

Continue to pay attention to your breathing and now focus on your out-breath. As you exhale, imagine that the out-breath carries with it and away from you any fears about speaking your truth; anything that blocks you from communicating with the world in an authentic way; every 'yes' when you meant to say 'no'; your shyness; guilt; and your need for gossip.

Now say, either out loud or in your head: 'I choose to speak my truth. I liberate myself from suffocating guilt. My words are magnets to attract genuine and clear energy into my life. I embrace my authentic voice and allow others' expression to be different from mine.' Take a few gentle breaths while reflecting on where you can respond to negativity with silence; breathe while listening to others; where you need to speak up; how you can engage more with your voice by singing or chanting; how you can move away from people who always make you feel guilty or impose their words onto you.

Now move your awareness to the third eye chakra in the middle of your forehead, the centre of your intuition and inner vision. Imagine that here you ignite a little twinkle of indigo-blue light. Focus on your in-breath, imagine the air smells of lavender, and draw your breath really deep down into this ball of light. Each time you do so it expands and the glow becomes brighter. The indigo-blue light creates a pulse of vibrant energy. Feel this energy. See the light flare and illuminate all the space in and around you with a bright indigo blue light as if the vast expanse of a midnight sky has opened around you. You're inside a bright sparkle of indigo-blue light.

Continue to pay attention to your breathing and now focus on your out-breath. As you exhale, imagine that the out-breath carries with it and away from you any negative self-image; any fears of being unable to find a solution to life's problems; anything that blocks your imagination or prevents you from a clear perception; and anything that silences your intuition.

Now say, either out loud or in your head: 'I have the ability to see the bigger picture and find a hidden perspective. I respect my intuition as my teacher. I am aligned with a limitless source of guidance. My imagination is a threshold towards the infinite pool of possibilities. It navigates me towards authentic choices.' Take a few gentle breaths while reflecting on where some gifts in your life came disguised as losses; who or what makes you doubt your intuition; how you can create a mood board for the life you'd like to attract and which resonates with your truth.

Finally, focus on the area just above your head that encircles the very crown of your head like a halo: the crown chakra. This is the centre of your consciousness and spirituality. Imagine that here you ignite a little twinkle of violet light. Focus on your in-breath, imagine the air smells of frankincense and draw your breath really deep down into this ball of light. Each time you do so it expands and the glow becomes brighter. The violet light creates a pulse of vibrant energy. Feel this energy. See the violet light flare and unfold like a large lotus flower with a thousand petals. Its petals illuminate all the space in and around you with a bright violet light. You're inside the beautiful lotus flower of violet light.

Continue to pay attention to your breathing and now focus on your out-breath. As you exhale, imagine that the out-breath carries with it and away from you everything that sabotages your faith; anything that makes you doubt the spiritual side of life; anyone who brainwashes you and your ego, cutting your connection with your higher self.

Now say, either out loud or in your head: 'I am who I am and I glory in that. I find bliss in my unique expression and in my loving and trusting connection with the Universe.' Take a few gentle breaths while reflecting on how you can make the world a better place; the legacy you want to leave behind; how you can find more time for mindful living and meditation; how you can practise gratitude to the Universe for even the smallest things.

When you're ready, gently bring your awareness back into the room, knowing that you're connected to the grounding energy of the Earth and are guided by the Universe. Take a deep breath and have a good stretch. Slowly stand up, legs slightly apart, with a straight back and strong posture, almost like a soldier standing to attention.

Once again, as you did at the beginning of this meditation, place one hand on your solar plexus and cover it with the other one, then say out loud, if possible while looking at your reflection in a mirror and using your mother tongue: 'My energy ID is activated. I am a magnet only for what is true to myself. I *own* my energy.'

. . . .

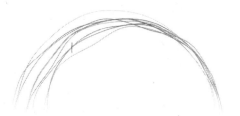

References

Prologue: Back to the Future – Hidden Risks to Our Wellbeing

1. Geltner, G., 2012. Public Health and the Pre-Modern City: A Research Agenda. *History Compass, 10*(3), 231-245.

2. Ibid. p.509–510

3. Ibid. p.510

4. Morgan, M., 2001. *National Identities and Travel in Victorian Britain.* Palgrave Macmillan UK.

Chapter 3: YOUnison

1. Young, L.J., and Wang, Z., 2004. The neurobiology of pair bonding. *Nature Neuroscience, 7* (10, 1048–1054).

2. Johnson, Z.V., and Young, L.J., 2015. Neurobiological mechanisms of social attachment and pair bonding. *Curr Opin Behav Sci, 3,* 38–44.

3. Leong, V., Byrne, E., Clackson, K., Georgieva, S., Lam, S., and Wass, S., 2017. Speaker gaze increases information coupling between infant and adult brains. Available at: <www.biorxiv.org/content/biorxiv/early/2017/09/16/108878.full.pdf> [accessed 11 April 2019].

4. Feldman, R., Magori-Cohen, R., Galili, G., Singer, M., and Louzoun, Y., 2011. Mother and infant coordinate heart rhythms through episodes

of interaction synchrony. *Infant Behavior and Development, 34*(4), 569–577.

5. Bowlby, J., 1969. *Attachment and Loss 1: Attachment.* New York: Basic Books.

6. Brown, M.R., 1982. Corticotropin-releasing factor: actions on the sympathetic nervous system and metabolism. *Endocrinology,* 111, 928–931.

7. Schore, A.N., 1994. *Affect Regulation and the Origin of the Self: The Neurobiology of Emotional Development.* Mahwah, NJ: Lawrence Eribaum.

8. Schore, A.N., 2001. The effects of early relational trauma on right-brain development, affect regulation and infant mental health. *Infant Mental Health Journal 22,* 1–2, 201–269.

9. Bowlby, J., 1973. *Attachment and Loss 2: Separation: Anxiety and Anger.* New York: Basic Books.

10. Marvin, R.S., 1977. An ethological-cognitive model for the attenuation of mother–child attachment behavior. In: T. M. Alloway et al (eds.), *Advances in the Study of Communication and Affect 3: Attachment Behavior.* New York: Plenum Press, 25–60.

11. Hamzei, F., Vry, M.S., Saur, D., Glauche, V., Hoeren, M., Mader, I., and Rijntjes, M., 2015. The dual-loop model and the human mirror neuron system: an exploratory combined fMRI and DTI study of the inferior frontal gyrus. *Cerebral Cortex, 26*(5). Available at: <https://academic.oup.com/cercor/article/26/5/2215/1754273.> [accessed 10 April 2019].

12. Hobson, H.M. and Bishop, D.V., 2016. Mu suppression – a good measure of the human mirror neuron system? *Cortex, 82.* Available at: <https://core.ac.uk/download/pdf/82008503.pdf> [accessed 11 April 2019].

13. Isbilir, E., Cakir, M., Cummins, F., and Ayaz, H., 2016. Investigating brain–brain interactions of a dyad using fNIR hyperscanning during joint sentence reading task. In: 3rd International Symposium on Brain Cognitive Science.

14. Verdiere, K.J, Roy, R.N., and Dehais, F., 2018. Detecting pilot's engagement using fNIRS connectivity features in an automated vs. manual landing scenario. *Frontiers in Human Neuroscience, 12*(6).

15. Hirsch, J., Zhang, X., Noah, J.A., and Ono, Y., 2017. Frontal temporal and parietal systems synchronize within and across brains during live eye-to-eye contact. *Neuroimage, 157*, 314–330.

16. Kodama, K., Tanaka, S., Shimizu, D., Hori, K., and Matsui, H., 2018. Heart rate synchrony in psychological counselling: a case study. *Psychology, 9*(07), 1858.

17. Mitkidis, P., McGraw, J.J., Roepstorff, A., and Wallot, S., 2015. Building trust: heart rate synchrony and arousal during joint action increased by public goods game. *Physiology & Behavior, 149*, 101–106.

18. Ferrer, E., and Helm, J.L., 2012. Dynamical systems modelling of physiological coregulation in dyadic interactions. *Int. J. Psychophysiol, 88*(3).

19. Helm, J.L., Sbarra, D., and Ferrer, E., 2012. Assessing cross-partner associations in physiological responses via coupled oscillator models. *Emotion, 12*(4), 748–762.

20. Kang, O., and Wheatley, T., 2017. Pupil dilation patterns spontaneously synchronize across individuals during shared attention. *Journal of Experimental Psychology: General, 146*(4), 569.

21. Garcia, A.M., and Ibáñez, A., 2014. Two-person neuroscience and naturalistic social communication: the role of language and linguistic variables in brain-coupling research. *Frontiers in Psychiatry, 5*, 214.

22. McGettigan, C., and Tremblay, P., 2018. Links between perception and production: examining the roles of motor and premotor cortices in understanding speech. In: S. Rueschemeyer and M. Gaskell (Eds.), *The Oxford Handbook of Psycholinguistics*, 306–334. Oxford, UK: Oxford University Press.

23. Wilson, S.M., Saygin, A.P., Sereno, M.I., and Iacoboni, M., 2004. Listening to speech activates motor areas involved in speech production. *Nature Neuroscience, 7*, 701–702.

24. Coupland, N., 2010. Accommodation theory. *Society and Language Use, 7*, 21–43.

25. Gijssels, T., Casasanto, L.S., Jasmin, K., Hagoort, P., and Casasanto, D., 2016. Speech accommodation without priming: the case of pitch. *Discourse Processes, 53*(4), 233–251.

26. Pedersen, S.B., 2015. *The cognitive ecology of human errors in emergency medicine: an interactivity-based approach.* PhD. University of Southern Denmark, Odense, DK.

27. Engert, V., Ragsdale, A.M., and Singer, T., 2018. Cortisol stress resonance in the laboratory is associated with inter-couple diurnal cortisol covariation in daily life. *Hormones and Behavior, 98*, 183–190.

28. Handlin, L., Hydring-Sandberg, E., Nilsson, A., Ejdebäck, M., Jansson, A., and Uvnäs-Moberg, K., 2015. Short-term interaction between dogs and their owners: effects on oxytocin, cortisol, insulin and heart rate – an exploratory study. *Anthrozoös, 24*(3), 301–315. DOI: 10.2752/17530 3711X13045914865385

29. Buttner, A.P., Thompson, B., Strasser, R., and Santo, J., 2015. Evidence for a synchronization of hormonal states between humans and dogs during competition. *Physiology & Behavior, 147*, 54–62.

30. Cunningham, K., 2017. *Hormonal synchronization between therapy dogs and handlers.* Paper presented at the 9th Annual Student Research and Creative Productivity Fair, Omaha, NE.

31. Miller, S.C., Kennedy, C.C., DeVoe, D.C., Hickey, M., Nelson, T., and Kogan, L., 2015. An examination of changes in oxytocin levels in men and women before and after interaction with a bonded dog. *Anthrozoös, 22*(1), 31–42. DO1: 10.2752/175303708X390455

32. Handlin, L., Nilsson, A., Ejdebäck, M., Hydbring-Sandberg, E., and Uvnäs-Moberg, K., 2015. Associations between the psychological characteristics of the human-dog relationship and oxytocin and cortisol levels. *Anthrozoös, 25*(2), 215–228. DOI: 10.2752/175303712 X13316289505468

33. McCraty et al., 2015. The Energetic Heart: Biolectromagnetic Interactions Within and Between People. Available at: <www.researchgate.net/publication/274451622_The_Energetic_Heart_Biolectromagnetic_Interactions_Within_and_Between_People> [accessed 28 May 2019].

Chapter 8: The Digital Layer of the Aura

1. Ghosn, R., Yahia-Cherif, L., Hugueville, L., Ducorps, A., Lemaréchal, J.D., Thuróczy, G., de Seze, R., and Selmaoui, B., 2015. Radiofrequency signals affect alpha band in resting electroencephalogram. *Journal of Neuropathy*, *113*(7). Available at: <www.physiology.org/doi/full/10.1152/jn.00765.2014> [accessed 11 April 2019].

2. Roggeveen, S., van Os, J., Viechtbauer, W., and Lousberg, R., 2015. EEG changes due to experimentally induced 3G mobile phone radiation. *PLoS ONE*, *10*(6), e0129496. Available at: <www.ncbi.nlm.nih.gov/pmc/articles/PMC4459698/> [accessed 11 April 2019].

3. Lv, B., Chen, Z., Wu, T., Shao, Q., Yan, D., Ma, L., and Xie, Y., 2014. The alteration of spontaneous low-frequency oscillations caused by acute electromagnetic fields exposure. *Clinical Neurophysiology*, *125*(2), 277–286.

4. Hung, C.S., Anderson, C., Horne, J.A., and McEvoy, P., 2007. Mobile phone 'talk-mode' signal delays EEG-determined sleep onset. *Neuroscience Letters*, *421*(1), 82–86.

5. Burgess, A.P., Fouquet, N.C., Seri, S., Hawken, M.B., Heard. A., Neasham, D., and Elliott, P., 2016. Acute exposure to Terrestrial Trunked Radio (TETRA) has effects on the electroencephalogram and electrocardiogram, consistent with vagal nerve stimulation. *Environmental Research*, *150*, 461–469.

6. Huss, A., van Eijsden, M., Guxens, M., Beekhuizen, J., van Strien, R., Kromhout, H., Vrijkotte, T., and Vermeulen, R., 2015. Environmental radio frequency electromagnetic fields exposure at home, mobile and cordless phone use, and sleep problems in 7-year-old children. *PLoS ONE*, *10*(10), e0139869.

7. Danker-Hopfe, H., Dorn, H., Bolz, T., Peter, A., Hansen, M.L., Eggert, T., and Sauter, C., 2016. Effects of mobile phone exposure (GSM 900 and WCDMA/UMTS) on polysomnography based sleep quality: an intra- and inter-individual perspective. *Environmental Research*, *145*, 50–60.

8. Mohammed, H.S., Fahmy, H.M., Radwan, N.M., and Elsayed, A.A., 2013. Non-thermal continuous and modulated electromagnetic radiation fields effects on sleep EEG of rats. *Journal of Advanced Research*, *4*(2), 181–187.

9.   Lustenberger, C., Murbach, M., Dürr, R., Schmid, M.R., Kuster, N., Achermann, P., and Huber, R., 2013. Stimulation of the brain with radio frequency electromagnetic pulses affects sleep-dependent performance improvement. *Brain Stimulation, 6*(5), 805–811.

10. Christensen, M.A., Bettencourt, L., Kaye, L., Moturu, S.T., Nguyen, K.T., Olgin, J.E., Pletcher, M.J., and Marcus, G.M., 2016. Direct measurements of smartphone screen-time: relationships with demographics and sleep. *PLoS ONE, 11*(11): e0165331. Available at: <https://journals.plos.org/plosone/article?id=10.1371/journal.pone.0165331> [accessed 10 April 2019].

11. Chak, K., and Leung, L., 2004. Internet addiction and internet use. *CyberPsychology & Behavior, 7*(5).

12. Bian, M., and Leung, L., 2014. Linking loneliness, shyness, smartphone addiction symptoms, and patterns of smartphone use to social capital. *Social Science Computer Review.*

13. Smetaniuk, P., 2014. A preliminary investigation into the prevalence and prediction of problematic cell phone use. *J Behav Addict, 3*(1), 41–53.

14. Kwon, M., Lee, J-Y., Won, W-Y., Park, J-W., Min, J-A., Hahn, C., et al, 2013. Development and validation of a smartphone addiction scale (SAS). *PLoS One, 8*(2), e56936. Available at: <https://journals.plos.org/plosone/article?id=10.1371/journal.pone.0056936> [accessed 11 April 2019].

Chapter 9: Digital Living Versus Digital Slavery

1.   Kramer, R.S.S., Weger, U.W., and Sharma, D., 2013. The effect of mindfulness meditation on time perception. *Consciousness and Cognition, 22*(3), 846–852.

2.   Ward, A.F., Duke, K., Gneezy, A., and Bos, M.W., 2017. Brain drain: the mere presence of one's own smartphone reduces available cognitive capacity. *Journal of the Association for Consumer Research, 2*(2).

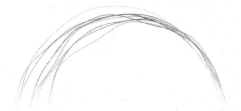

Index

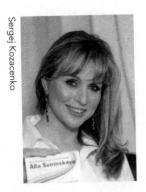

Sergej Kozacenko

About the Author

Alla Svirinskaya is a medically trained, fifth-generation energy healer who is now considered one of the world's top experts in holistic wellness. She has acted as a senior consultant to leading spas around the world, including the iconic Chiva-Som in Thailand.

Alla's books, *Energy Secrets* and *Your Secret Laws of Power*, have become international bestsellers and been translated into 16 languages. Alla is famed for her systematic, no-nonsense approach to the healing process, and counts numerous celebrity and royal clients among the thousands of people she has helped.

www.allasvirinskaya.com

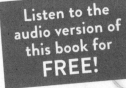